Ditch THE Diet

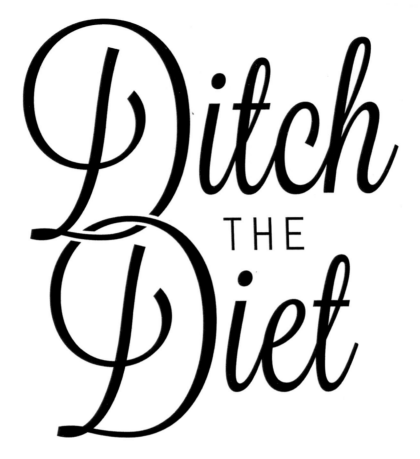

HOW TO
RECLAIM YOUR HEALTH
AND ENJOY FOOD

Connie,
I always enjoy
our chats when I
stop by the church.
Thank you for all you
do. for the love
of food,
Julie

JULIE SIEJA SATTERFEAL, MS, RDN, LD

TRIPLE BRAIDED, LLC

Ditch the Diet: How to Reclaim Your Health and Enjoy Food
ISBN: 978-0-9992459-0-3
First Printing

Published in the United States of America by:

Triple Braided, LLC
710 Andrew Jackson Way
Huntsville, AL 35801
www.triplebraided.com

To order a copy of this book please visit:
www.triplebraided.com

The information provided in this book is intended to help guide and educate those wishing to know more about nutrition and diet choices. It is not a substitute for individualized nutrition and/or healthcare services. In no way is this book intended to replace the advice given to you by your own physician. Nor is the author or Triple Braided, LLC responsible for any specific health or allergy needs that may require medical supervision and are not liable for any damages or negative consequences from any treatment, action, application or preparation, to any person reading or following the information in this book. Information in this book is general and is offered with no guarantees on the part of the author or Triple Braided, LLC. The author disclaims all liability in connection with the use of this book.

Dedication

This book is dedicated to my husband,
whose unwavering belief in me
has been my rock and sustaining force.

Contents

Acknowledgments

THANK YOU TO my editor, Lady Smith, the first person to read my work, and whose keen mind and extraordinary abilities were integral in the development and presentation of my ideas. Your advice and feedback made all the difference and kept me focused and accountable. Thank you to Steven Jackson for answering my random questions when I needed a reliable resource and handling the technicalities as well as the strategies of marketing and promotions. Thanks to Thrive Creative Group for taking my graphic visions and making them a reality.

Thank you to my clients for trusting me with some fragile pieces of your being, and for being willing to take a leap of faith and set aside the "comfort" of dieting. The opportunity to work with each of you is what gave this book purpose. To the participants and attendees of my challenges, group programs, seminars, and all of you who show up, thank you for the validation, your time, and your efforts. I also appreciate the great women of St. Mark's Lutheran Church who have made a deliberate effort to be supportive of my book writing endeavor.

I am grateful to the very special people willing to read this book and provide your encouraging feedback: Brianna Sieja, Mardell Wilson, Dixie Bailey, and Tim Sieja. Your thoughts worked to build me up and gave me the courage to release this project to the public. And to my mother, Kathy Sieja, who not only read my work but also contributed her expertise to this book, nothing would have been possible without you. Thank you to my brother, Andy Sieja, for helping me untangle the legal jargon and keeping me on the level. And I am grateful to my dad, Don Sieja, for your humor and allowing me to tell stories on you. To all my family and my friends who bolster and encourage me and continue to validate my book's content as important, your commitment was especially powerful each time I questioned myself and my purpose. With all of your individual talents and gifts I felt as if God placed each of you in my path at exactly the moment I needed you most. I especially appreciate my running buddies (Brianna Sieja, Erin Cobb, Angela Rawls, Brooke Edmondson), Lara Sieja, Kimberly Bellis, Marcus Singleton, Janell Zesinger, Jane Argentina, Amy Jackson, and each of you dear friends that I have not listed by name. You know who you are.

My children, Sesalie, Noah, and Kinsley, bring meaning to my life in ways I could never have imagined and ways that are new every morning; you inspire me with the gifts of who you are and your unique perspectives on the world. I am so grateful to be your mom and have the opportunity to make you dinner each night—even if I do grumble about it occasionally. Thank you for your unconditional love. It is everything. And to my husband, Craig Satterfeal, my rock and grounding support: you knew I would get here even when I doubted, and it has made all the difference.

Preface

I'LL NEVER FORGET an evening in early 2004 when, as a young mother, I found myself on the floor of a local bookstore, exhausted and frustrated to tears. In front of me was a shelf with about 800 books on how to get your baby to sleep—each with advice that seemed to contradict the other. I had a 1-year-old and an infant with separate sets of sleeping dilemmas—and I was getting no sleep as a result. I remember thinking, "What is the *right* answer? None of these scenarios fits my circumstances. I wish I could get advice from someone I trust and whose parenting style and ideas align with mine." Then and there, in my moment of personal crisis, I had a profound aha moment related to my profession. "This," I thought, "is how my discouraged clients feel about the truckloads of diets and contradictory nutrition information that is everywhere! No wonder they are in a puddle of tears by the time they show up at my office."

Thus—after I pulled myself up off the store floor—began my crusade to determine the best way to help people navigate the diet industry. As it turns out, the real solution is to completely Ditch the Diet.

You may never have had a meltdown in your neighborhood bookstore, but do you feel overwhelmed by the chatter about the latest diets and confused about where to turn for answers? Do you ever wish for someone to simply tell you what to do? You are not alone. And, unfortunately, those desperate feelings and deep frustrations are ripe conditions for a fad diet to swoop in with a pretend solution. Diets give us what we think we need; however, they usually lead us into further frustration, despair, and oftentimes weight gain.

Through my years of study and working with people, I have found some common threads among dieters. These tendencies can be summed up in the "Evolution of a Dieter" diagram found in the front of this book. I created this diagram as a one-stop overview to depict some of the complications that happen with dieting. It shows how the intricacies of our brain intertwine with our body to make dieting a losing battle.

In the coming chapters we are going to discuss first the flaws that make diets ineffective and then the strategies for how to Ditch the Diet—forever. We will cover practical, manageable ways to lead a healthy and happy life that is filled with enjoyable food. We all want to be healthy and to feel good. I would guess that even those of you who have never dieted before still have questions about good nutrition, and get confused about all the mixed messages out there. "Is gluten bad for you, and should we limit how much we eat for general health? What about fat and cholesterol? Should I be eating more protein?"

In the chapters focusing on solutions, we will let The Pyramid to Healthy Eating guide us. I created this pyramid to depict the concepts that are foundational to a healthy relationship with food: Eat Mindfully, Allow Yourself to Eat, and Accept Your Body. In turn, those concepts will make it possible for you to Eat Nutritionally by learning how to Create Lasting Habits. My hope is that each reader can gain some insight and answers about food, nutrition, eating, and weight—and that you never find yourself in an exasperated and confused panic about what to eat. Food is one of the great pleasures of life. So let's learn how to Ditch the Diet, regain our health, and enjoy food once and for all.

Chapter 1
The Definition of Dieting and Why to Stop

Affirmation: I love myself.

As A WELLNESS DIETITIAN, my life is saturated with the subject of dieting. I am writing this book because I really want that to change, and for you to Ditch the Diet forever and for good. I have heard so many personal stories detailing the diets my clients and friends have been on and the feelings and patterns that have gone along with them. When someone tells me that they have been on *all* the diets, it is amazing to me how similar that person's experience is to the many other lifelong dieters I have spoken with. They generally feel very alone, but I'm here to tell you that they are not. I hope that we can shed light on the dieting mindset, which has become a perpetual struggle for more people than ever.

In conversations with clients, when I describe some of the typical thought processes that accompany a diet, people are floored because I'm usually describing something they have experienced. I have found that dieters' experiences are similar not because of the diets they have chosen to follow but because of the very fact that they *are dieting*. If you are reading this book and have been on a diet before, I have a feeling your story will fit right in. And if you have never dieted before, I imagine you will recognize loved ones in the scenarios I present, and you may discover a new way of understanding what they are going through.

Just what are diets anyway? In American culture it seems that diets have become a list of rules about how much and what foods to eat and which foods to avoid, all with the ultimate goal of losing weight. Yet unfortunately, what seems like—and is promoted as—a very straightforward concept is actually anything but straightforward or simple. Even the definition of the word *diet* is fraught with problems. The primary definition according to *Merriam-Webster* mentions "habitual nourishment" as well as "a regimen of eating and drinking sparingly so as to reduce one's weight." The origin of the word comes from the Greek *diaita*, which means "manner of living," and *diaitasthai*, "to lead one's life." All of this provides insight, but it is the secondary meaning of *diet* that really blows me away: "something provided or experienced repeatedly (a *diet* of Broadway shows and nightclubs)." With this definition focusing on repetition, we really get to the heart of the matter. Diets, as we know them, are so wholly ineffective that they have given rise to this second meaning—a slang use of the term that encompasses its dysfunction. If a diet must be experienced repeatedly, then in fact it ultimately did not or does not work. And thus we have a culture of chronic dieting.

We all know that famous definition of insanity that Albert Einstein may (or may not) have coined: "doing the same thing over and over again and expecting different results." Yet somehow we don't recognize the insanity inherent in dieting. I would assume that is because most people don't see dieting as doing the same thing over and over again. With each "new" diet, they think they are trying a different course of action. Now pay attention, as this is the part we have to wrap our minds around: It does not matter that every diet you try consists of different food restrictions, because that is not why a diet ultimately fails. Diet success is not going to be attained by finding the "right" diet. Even if you lost weight on a certain diet, it was not successful if you eventually gained the weight back. And finding a new diet is not the answer you should be looking for. You want to find a solution that is not a diet. You say, "I know, I know, I need to change my lifestyle, and I know what I need to do. I just have to do it." Based on what I've learned from working with clients over the years, chances are your idea of "changing your lifestyle" is actually going on a diet. Truly changing your lifestyle does not happen overnight, nor does it result in fast weight loss. Therefore, if your lifestyle change comes with a weight-loss goal for the end of the month, then I have news for you: it's a diet.

Diets are extremely complicated, so we will spend the first half of this book exploring the full scope of the definition of dieting, as well as how diets affect most people. Dieting is never a simple scientific equation, despite what a certain plan might try to tell you. Diets will generally lead you into a dangerous cycle which I have come to call the Dieting Trifecta. You'll learn much more about the Dieting Trifecta in chapter 4, but for now, let's look at some of the red flags signaling that you may be headed for dieting disaster. Most diets incorporate one or all of these red flags:

Dieting Trifecta Red Flags

- Plans that eliminate entire food groups and promise rapid weight loss.
- Requiring adherence to strict calorie deficits for any length of time.
- Eating only a few selected foods for any period of time.
- Ergogenic aids, energy aids, diet pills, and quick fixes for the purpose of weight loss.

If any of these red flags are pieces of your current lifestyle, strategies you've tried before, or things you think you should be doing, then keep reading. I want you to free yourself from the bondage of diets, and the internal strife, self-loathing, and shame that they inevitably create.

Diets feel as if they are the answer to improving your health or weight, but they are not. Diets are moving you in the wrong direction and creating the exact problems you are trying to fix.

I have learned much about the thought patterns of dieters through my years of study and working with people as a registered dietitian. And I have discovered some common tendencies, which I used to create the "Evolution of a Dieter" diagram found in the front of this book. This diagram depicts some of the complications that happen with dieting, particularly the way our thoughts interact with our physiology to cause a dangerous dieting cycle. The following three chapters will cover each section of this diagram in more detail. Once we finish looking closely at the perils of dieting, we will dive into some solutions. We will explore exactly what to do after you Ditch the Diet. Using a Pyramid to Healthy Eating, we will work our way through the foundational steps that are necessary to move out of dieting and into a life filled with health and enjoyment of food. Let's turn the page and start our journey toward discovering solutions that work for you.

Chapter 2
The Evolution of a Dieter

Affirmation: I am more than this.

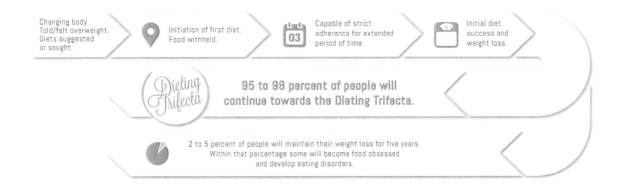

Changing body. Told/felt overweight. Diets suggested or sought. → Initiation of first diet. Food withheld. → Capable of strict adherence for extended period of time. → Initial diet success and weight loss.

Dieting Trifecta — 95 to 98 percent of people will continue towards the Dieting Trifecta.

2 to 5 percent of people will maintain their weight loss for five years. Within that percentage some will become food obsessed and develop eating disorders.

A PERSON'S FIRST DIET may happen at any age—during the preteen years, in high school or college, when trying to take off postpartum baby weight, or anytime at all. Regardless of when it occurs, that first diet often sets into motion a predictable pattern of events. The initiation of the first diet may happen for a variety of reasons: normal developmental changes occur in your body that make you feel different or uncomfortable; a parent, doctor, or friend says you are overweight; you buy in to societal and media messages glorifying one body type and equating it with beauty and happiness. I call this pattern of events and the ensuing physical, emotional, and intellectual consequences the "Evolution of a Dieter." I believe the results, depending upon the individual, can be damaging no matter when the onset of the first diet, though it may have more lasting consequences the earlier it happens (see the end of this chapter for more on dieting during adolescence).

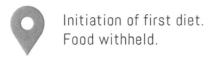

Initiation of first diet.
Food withheld.

The Evolution of a Dieter begins with the initiation of that first diet, which, for many of us, can be very energizing and exciting. The diet is a new plan with the prospect of making all our dreams come true. No matter how vain it may seem or how unlikely it is to gain true happiness by weighing less, we convince ourselves that everything else in life will become more manageable when we are thinner. That idea gives us the excitement and motivation to embark on a new eating regimen. We clean out the pantry of anything not on the plan, buy different and "healthy" foods, find new recipes for all our meals, and give ourselves pep talks about how great this will make us feel. We have delusions of grandeur that we can do anything for a short period of time, after which we can go back to life as we know it.

 Capable of strict adherence for extended period of time.

With all of this energy and motivation, a typical adult is generally capable of strictly adhering to the diet and its calorie restrictions for an extended period of time. (Remember this, because dieters certainly do. The fact that dieters are able to successfully adhere to that very first diet for an extended time will continue to torture and eat away at them in the future when they are less able to do so. This contributes to why many of us try diets over and over again, and it plays into the self-loathing and frustration we feel when we are unable to adhere as well and attain the same level of success down the road.)

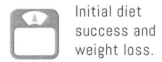 Initial diet success and weight loss.

Continuing the evolution, as a result of adhering to the strict calorie restrictions of whatever diet plan is chosen, the dieter has initial diet success and weight loss. Take note of the phrase "whatever diet plan is chosen." This is a huge point of confusion. Though people make all kinds of assumptions about which diets work for them, it is not necessarily a particular diet or the elimination of certain foods that make it "work." This diet seems to work simply because this diet is the first one. Not only does the dieter start off with a full reservoir of energy and motivation that make it possible to stick to food restrictions, but the body is also more capable of weight loss in that initial attempt. As time goes on, willpower loses to the power of human nature's hunger. Any food restrictions become more difficult with each new diet attempt.

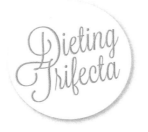 95 to 98 percent of people will continue towards the Dieting Trifecta.

This is the point in the Evolution of a Dieter at which 95 to 98 percent of dieters will continue toward the Dieting Trifecta, the black hole of dieting described in detail in chapter 4, in which a vicious cycle of weight regain, weight loss, weight regain plus more, ensues. The other 2 to 5 percent of dieters will maintain their weight loss for five years, the period of time that has been deemed by the medical community to indicate "successful weight loss."

This Evolution of a Dieter I've described—a person evolving into a chronic dieter—is based on what I have witnessed firsthand with clients and seen in the research that has looked at dieting and weight regain. Yet the progression is not an absolute, following exactly the same path. Different diets produce different results because of the foods they include or restrict, and physiology and human nature respond differently as well. This is one of the reasons that we see new fad diet trends come and go. The biggest shift in my lifetime has probably been the transition of fad diets from low-/no-fat to low-carbohydrate and high-protein. (See chapter 8 for how and why that shift happened, and why both fads are poor solutions to healthy eating.)

Dieting is a big industry, and companies are making coin on the backs of desperate people that will try anything. And people are desperate to try anything because they have been told they are unhealthy, unattractive, and weak-minded if they carry extra pounds. Society discriminates against overweight individuals and encourages assumptions about their lifestyles, insinuating, for example, that they are lazy, have no self-control, and must be indulging in massive portions of junk food. In my experience, the chronic dieter is the absolute opposite of those stereotypes. Chronic dieters find themselves in the dieting predicament precisely because they know how to be successful: they have tried and succeeded at multiple drastic weight-loss attempts over and over again. Each short-term success makes them more likely to go back and try it all again.

Despite a growing awareness that diets are harmful, diet gurus and solicitors continue to proliferate and gain followers, for two primary reasons:

1. Diets offer quick results, satisfying human nature's need for immediate gratification.
2. Weight regain and diet failure are always internalized. Dieters blame themselves, and then go back for more with new resolve to do better.

This repeating cycle—or, more aptly, this train wreck waiting to happen—can begin at various points in life, yet I've noticed some common trends in my years working with different people. One trend is that most adults dealing with extra weight and a history of repeat dieting tell me that they went on their first diet as a child, preteen, or teenager. Let's take a look at adolescence and how a changing body, the young mind, and societal messages can impact a young person embarking on a diet.

A natural point for personal body self-awareness happens at the onset of puberty, when the body begins to change at a more rapid pace. We all grow at different rates and in different ways, but this stage in our development can be particularly jarring as the physical distinctions among people become more apparent. Consider, for example, two 12-year-old girls who have similar builds at the end of their sixth-grade school year: they are the same height, both flat chested with a straight figure and slight frame. They come back after summer break to begin their seventh-grade year, and one girl looks exactly the same while the other has developed some breasts, her hips have begun to broaden, and her face is a bit fuller with a few blemishes here and there. Then consider how varied these distinctions can be among peers when pubescent changes begin for some as early as 8 years old and don't start for others until the teen years. Given that the average age of puberty is about 12, we can all remember what a diverse group middle-schoolers can be!

So many changes are happening during the adolescent years, and the outward, physical ones are just the tip of the iceberg. It is difficult to go from being a kid that loves playing and acting silly to a preteen who wants to fit in with social groups and seem confident and cool. Adolescents are trying to figure out what their interests are and where they fit in, while adults are beginning to expect more mature behavior and schoolwork is becoming more important and time-consuming. Meanwhile, each child is experiencing a powerful dose of emotions that are all over the spectrum: anger and irritability, embarrassment, shame, anxiety, unbridled excitement, joy, fear. Adolescence brings so much change, and so little control.

Now mix all of this with body image. Some preteens skate right through this stage with no body image issues, but for others adolescence can be a critical point. Not only can physical insecurities be self-imposed, but they can also be instigated by friends and, unfortunately and more commonly, by parents.

During this time, as parents watch these body changes taking place in their child, they can become unnecessarily concerned for their child's health. In response, and with diets becoming an accepted norm, many parents put their children on diets, restrict their food, and put a large focus on eating. This is an inappropriate course of action, and can lay a foundation that leads to lifelong dieting, subsequent weight issues, and even other serious health implications.

In this and other instances, parents may also transfer some of their own eating and weight baggage to their children. Not only do kids see and hear their parents' perceptions of and feelings about their own bodies, but they internalize those messages in relation to themselves. If the adults in their lives are dieting, children pick up on it. When the adults they look up to criticize their own bodies, children will in turn begin to question theirs as well.

For all of these reasons, adolescence or childhood is often when someone goes on, or is put on, their first diet. And this first diet can set into motion a predictable and troubling pattern of events. Though the results of dieting can be damaging no matter the age, the delicacy of childhood—along with the lack of control a child has in terms of food intake—adds important dimensions to the problem. The result can be absolutely heartbreaking.

Children are not going to find diets energizing or exciting. The experience for them is likely to be physically tortuous and mentally degrading and shaming. Additionally, children are going to resist hunger, which leads them to problem-solve: hiding or stockpiling food, and overeating at times when the guardian of the diet is not around. In other words, children that are placed on a diet will enter the Dieting Trifecta sooner.

So, now to the big question: what are we supposed to do when we or our children are labeled as overweight, and we are being told by society, peers, family, and/or health-care professionals to lose weight? The answer is not simple, nor is it the same for everyone. Because we are individuals with diverse histories, genetics, and personal stories, the plan of action we choose will certainly vary. But, after we come to understand some basics about metabolism and the Dieting Trifecta, covered in the next two chapters, I will provide some plans of action, plans that incorporate foundational eating and nutrition principles, and effective paths toward eating competence and a healthy body.

Chapter 3
What Does Metabolism Really Mean?

Affirmation: I was made for this.

AS WE'RE TRYING to understand the patterns and pitfalls of dieting, let's take a closer look at metabolism. The term is thrown around a lot, but what does metabolism really mean? Even I struggle with defining it. Just recently, my 15-year-old daughter asked me to please explain it to her. Some of her school friends had told her she must have a "fast metabolism," and she wanted to know what that means and whether it is true. If you are familiar with teens, then you know that they expect quick, concise answers or they will lose interest and move on—or maybe that is just my fast-moving, free-spirited oldest child. Unfortunately, despite my nutrition expertise and experience, I failed on the quick, concise answer. I started with a mangled, "Well, we are all different and metabolism refers to how our body uses energy or calories, and I would guess you have a good metabolism … blah blah [fumbling over words here]." I eventually referenced my handy chart, but you'd think I could have nailed the answer to my daughter's question without having to get help from my own guidebook. In my defense, it is a complicated subject. So, take two—with you, my readers!

As we launch into a few of the basics related to metabolism, it is important to consider our individuality, and because of that there is no set formula for determining or controlling metabolism. There are lots of formulas out there, and some of us can geek out with science all day long trying to find *the* one. But I encourage you to remember that each human is more than a scientific calculation. The physical and emotional results of dieting show how damaging it can be to turn humans into robots with prescribed formulas to fix our problems. So, we are going to look at some formulas related to metabolism, under the condition that you remember that these are simply estimates, and they fluctuate from person to person depending upon many individual factors.

Our metabolism is made up of three main components: Resting Metabolic Rate (RMR), Physical Activity Level (PAL), and the Thermic Effect of Feeding (TEF). If you flip back to the Evolution of a Dieter diagram in the front of the book, you will see these three components of metabolism listed toward the bottom of the graphic. Throughout this chapter, we will go into more detail about each component and dispel some common myths associated with metabolism.

1. Resting Metabolic Rate (RMR)

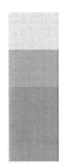

Resting Metabolic Rate (RMR) ★

Accounting for around 50-75% of the calories that we burn, this part of our metabolism is responsible for many of the tasks our bodies do to keep us alive and running like, breathing, blinking, regulating our temperature, pumping blood...etc.

When you diet your RMR plummets! Your body will conserve calories by slowing down!

The Resting Metabolic Rate is the approximate amount of calories our bodies burn to keep us alive. Notice the very large percentage associated with this component. That indicates we have very little control over this large chunk of our metabolism. We were created to do some stuff, and our body wants to keep us alive and moving and efficient.

Here's a peek into one of the physical effects of diets: you may be at the top of the RMR percentage, with your body burning 75 percent of the total calories you consume on its own internal business. Then you cut your calories way back for a few weeks in order to drop a few pounds, and in response your body decides to run a tighter ship. It's going to become more efficient and do the same job on fewer calories. So maybe now it uses only 60 percent of the calories you consume doing its own internal business. That's a significant change. #ThingsJustGotReal

2. Physical Activity Level (PAL)

Physical Activity Level (PAL) ★

Accounting for around 10-30% of our total metabolism this is the calorie burning that is created by the amount of physical activity that we have/engage in daily.

Increasing your activity will NOT offset the slowing of your RMR metabolism that results from dieting.

I love the acronym "PAL" for this component of metabolism because you should think of physical activity as your "pal"! Your Physical Activity Level will determine what percentage of the calories you consume will be burned by this part of your metabolism. Our PAL means that our body is using calories even when we are not specifically exercising. It includes the differences between working a desk job or waiting tables, how active we are when awake versus asleep, and variations in muscle mass, as muscle is metabolically active and having more muscle thus helps burn more calories.

I'm aware of a common myth when it comes to Physical Activity Level. The myth many dieters fall prey to is the belief that they can make up for the slowed metabolism caused from dieting by increasing their exercise. But that will help only to a certain degree. The reality is that cutting calories and increasing physical activity affect two different metabolic systems, so trying to offset one with the other is an ineffective option and a dangerous pitfall for dieters.

3. Thermic Effect of Feeding (TEF)

Thermic Effect of Feeding (TEF) ★

Accounting for around 5-15% of our total metabolism this is the calorie burning that is created in processing the food that we eat.

Skipping meals decreases opportunities for calorie burning, but you will burn muscle to get that needed energy.

The Thermic Effect of Feeding basically means that the body burns calories while processing calories. Every time we eat, our body has a whole lot of work to do, and it requires energy. There are the basics of chewing and swallowing, not to mention all the enzymatic reactions involved with the process of digestion. Then there is the energy required for nutrient absorption and the movement of food particles through our anatomy, as well as additional hormonal and cellular involvement. This thermic effect is another piece of our metabolism that we compromise with dieting and food restriction. Of course, the amount of calories burned while processing most foods does not come close to the amount of calories in those foods. Yet even so, frequently skipped meals and severely depressed calorie intake will have a significant impact on metabolism.

Quite often, I see people conceding this component of metabolism when it comes to breakfast. Breakfast seems to be a popular meal to try to cut calories on, and I can understand why. Here are a few of my theories:

1. Many people are not hungry for breakfast. Shouldn't they take advantage of that rare gift of appetite suppression and save calories since the appetite will come back with a vengeance later?

2. Many claim that eating breakfast makes them hungrier. If they skip breakfast, they can make it to lunch, yet when they eat breakfast they feel ravished by midmorning.

3. Mornings can be a hectic time. Skipping breakfast is an easy way to save time, especially if they're not hungry anyway.
4. With all the distractions of a busy morning, this is one of the rare occasions when food is not at the forefront of the mind.

I'd like to counter these breakfast-skipping justifications by paying attention to the Thermic Effect of Feeding:

1. Our resting metabolism has slowed overnight while we are sleeping, but it picks up when we wake and begin moving; when we eat breakfast, it picks up even more. By breaking the fast with breakfast, we provide our body with the energy it is waiting for to shift into high gear for the day. When we skip breakfast, we are not giving our body that opportunity for optimizing our metabolism.
2. By breaking the fast with a small, low-calorie breakfast that is limited in variety, we give ourselves just enough food to get our metabolism moving and start burning calories, but we will be hungry again in short order. A couple of options to fix this are to either have a larger, more sustainable breakfast or prepare for another small second breakfast. Both options will provide the nourishment our body needs, and will actually set us up for better hunger management at lunch and all day long.
3. Breakfast could take a significant amount of time, but it doesn't have to. Plan ahead or choose a quick option—because breakfast is that important. Skipping breakfast is a catalyst for a day of physical and emotional food disruptions.
4. When we eat a hearty breakfast, we won't think about food all day long the way that dieters do, because we are less hungry.

Genetics

This brings us to another factor related to metabolism and body type/shape that is even less formulaic yet an important piece of our overall discussion. We can consider this factor a fourth piece of metabolism although it encapsulates that and so much more. This factor is genetics. Our genetics will impact approximately 5 percent of our calorie burning. That means that from birth some of us burn more calories than others, for reasons unrelated to the three components of metabolism already discussed. So that "fast metabolism" my daughter asked me about is actually a thing. Naturally, the other three components we discussed will also contribute to her overall fast metabolism, but she may have a genetic booster to boot.

It is also estimated that 70 percent or more of our body type/shape is determined by our genetics. That means that our shape probably resembles the shape of one of our parents because of the genes they passed on to us—more than any habits they might have passed on as well. This is not to say that environment and nurture have nothing to do with our body shape, but they are not the main piece of the puzzle. We will come back to this concept again when we discuss the validity of weight charts.

Now that you are armed with a basic understanding of metabolism, we can move forward and address the role these physical aspects of metabolism play in the overall picture of dieting.

Chapter 4
The Dieting Trifecta

Affirmation: I am worthy of love.

I HAVE SPENT YEARS giving examples to my private-practice clients of all the ways that diets harm people. As I offer examples, I always have to back up to explain the progression of the dieting cycle, and how the body's physical reaction is only one component of the problem. Diets also mess with a person's head—both the intellectual part of the brain that is logically studying the biology, and the emotional part of the brain that is trying to make sense of feelings and preserve sanity. The way the intellectual mind and the emotional mind react then combines with the physical body, creating a whole new entity.

 Intellectual Mind   **Emotional Mind**   **Physical Body**

Ultimately, we have three dimensions coming together to create a dangerous combination. I have termed this the Dieting Trifecta, which is essentially a black hole or the Bermuda Triangle for dieters. Hitting the "trifecta" often means you've achieved a perfect series of three, maybe winning three major tennis tournaments, for example, or snagging three major Hollywood awards. The Dieting Trifecta is also a perfect threesome—but with nothing but negative results. When you become a chronic dieter, your intellectual mind, your emotional mind, and your physical body together create a dangerous cycle you can't escape. They lead you to a black hole where approximately 97 percent of all dieters end up, along with all the pounds they have lost and eventually regained. If you have dieted, lost weight, gained it back again, and dieted again, then you are probably there. Once you are in the Dieting Trifecta, you cannot escape by dieting. You just can't. You want to, and you will keep trying to, and society will tell you to, but you will fail. To escape the Dieting Trifecta, you must stop dieting.

Let's walk through the three dimensions that come together to create the Dieting Trifecta: the intellectual mind, the emotional mind, and the physical body. The Dieting Trifecta often begins with an intellectual approach to the diet, then includes how our psyche/mind reacts emotionally to dieting, and finally incorporates what is happening biologically and how our body physically handles the diet (including many of the metabolism factors we learned about in chapter 3). It tends to be a cycle that impacts the intellectual mind, the emotional mind, and the body—and then starts over again with the intellectual mind. With each cycle, the results are slightly different and potentially more harmful.

Because everyone is different, the timeframes of the cycle will fluctuate, as will the order in which they occur. As you read about them, you may find some of these examples to be spot on, while others may not be anything you recognize. Overall, this Dieting Trifecta scenario is a compilation of the messages that I hear and see repeatedly in my consultations with clients. Take it as a whole and understand that the concept is universal yet variable.

We are now picking up with what happens at the *end* of a diet. If you turn to the diagram of the Evolution of a Dieter, which can be found at the front of your book and unfolded to follow along, we are a third of the way down on the left with the words "The Thought Processes of the Three Dimensions." It is at this point that the dieter has gone on a fad diet and has successfully lost weight.

Cycle 1

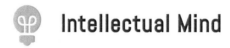

Intellectual Mind

Following mainstream messages that this is pure physiology and logical science. Eat less and lose weight, then transition to 'normal' calorie level.

I've lost the weight, now I can go back to a normal healthy diet, well rounded but not so restrictive.

It all starts in the **intellectual mind**. The world has told us repeatedly that losing weight is simply a matter of creating a calorie deficit: calories in versus calories out. It makes complete sense, and so all we need to do is eat less and exercise more, suffer for a short time feeling hungry and deprived of tasty food until the weight is off, and then go back to more moderate eating to maintain the new weight. We come to the end of the diet with a host of intellectual beliefs, most based on what we have been told:

- o We believe that before this diet, we acted as terrible gluttons and major overeaters, which led us to gain the weight in the first place.
- o We believe that, because we used to eat desserts and fried foods and cheese and chips, this weight gain was a predictable outcome.
- o We believe that our weight was the natural consequence for something we did wrong.

o   We also believe that, once we have finished our highly restrictive diet and lost all our "extra" pounds, we can transition back to a "normal, well-rounded, healthy diet," a diet where we are going to be much more careful about all those "bad" foods that caused our weight gain in the first place, but not so restrictive that we are hungry all the time like we were during the diet.

The problem with these beliefs is that many of them are wrong, and for a variety of reasons.

First, most weight is gained over a long period of time, insidiously sneaking up by an extra pound or two each year. Five years later, you're up a size, and then another size five years after that. Those few additional pounds per year are not the result of gluttony. They are little extras here and there: medication side effects, for instance, or added calories from meals eaten in restaurants (a much more common practice in modern times, due to the busy lives we lead and the convenience restaurants provide).

Second, as we age we lose muscle mass and our metabolism slows down. This can really be insidious because, as creatures of habit, we continue to pour ourselves the same size bowl of cereal even though our body may not need as much as we get older. We ought to listen to our bodies and eat mindfully—and we will learn how later, in chapter 7—but we tend to eat as we always have, and then blame ourselves for it later.

Additionally, we cannot forget that other factors such as increased stress and lack of sleep (unfortunately, now badges of honor in our society) are big contributors to the increasing size of our waistlines. All these factors and more play a part in our weight, but we convince ourselves—intellectually—that it is a simple situation that can be rectified by calorie counting.

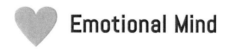 **Emotional Mind**

Want to relax and enjoy food after all the hard work and restrictions.

Yes, I did it! Now I can eat some of the things I love again...skinny people eat dessert right?

While our intellectual mind has logically explained the scientific reasons this diet has worked, our **emotional mind** adds a few tweaks and justifications. After being so good for so long on the highly restrictive diet, it becomes time to kick back, relax, and enjoy some of our favorite foods. "I'm not going to overdo it; I'm just going to have some of my favorite things that were not permissible on the weight-loss diet. Just look at all my skinny friends. They eat yummy foods and have never had a weight problem. I only had a weight problem because I really overdid it for a long time. I'm going to be more moderate this time around." Again, let us be reminded that there was no real "overdoing it" that led to the initial weight gain (or what may be merely a perceived weight gain). For most people it is a compilation of the factors previously addressed: genetics, normal developmental body changes, slowed metabolism with age and diets, processed food supply, putting on weight over a long period of time, a new cultural norm of eating out, increased stress and decreased sleep, and busy schedules. The dieter's emotional mind is trying to find a balance between enjoying some treats and still being nourished with healthy foods.

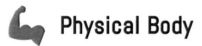

Physical Body

> Resting metabolism (RMR) has slowed down in response to restricted calories. Even small calorie increases can equal weight gain. ★
>
> Yes, finally food! Slow down, be more efficient, and store energy for the next famine.

While all the above thoughts are swirling in different areas of the dieter's mind, let's consider what is happening to the **physical body**. The diet created an initial crash in calories, which shocked the system and caught the body off-guard. The resulting weight loss has occurred in vehement opposition to what the inner workings of the physical body want to happen. In fact, it is a complete fail for the body. The body will take precautions, gradually, for drastic loss of body mass not to happen again. The first cycle of the Trifecta may produce one Physical Body Precaution, while each successive dieting cycle leads to additional physical precautions—each more damaging than the last, as we will see.

Physical Precaution 1: The Resting Metabolic Rate (RMR) slows down. Flip back to the metabolism explanation in chapter 3 for a quick refresher on what that means. Your body is not burning as many calories as it did pre-diet. Translation: As a post-diet 150-pound person, you can't eat as much food with the same result as you could when you were a pre-diet/never-dieted 150-pound person.

As all this happens in the mind and in the body, time passes and the weight slowly comes back on. The dieter considers another diet, and starts the cycle all over again, with slightly different and more damaging consequences.

Cycle 2

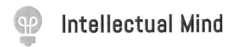 **Intellectual Mind**

Time to get back on another diet and keep close tabs on calories.

Did it before, will do it again. It won't affect my metabolism because I'll increase my exercise (PAL).

After some or most of the weight returns, the **intellectual mind** tells you it is time to do this thing again. Logically, this next new diet should not be too tough. Just watch the calories like last time. We believe we can be diligent, make a detailed plan of what to eat, and stick to it. Maybe we believe it's also time to increase exercise in order to prevent the decrease in calories from affecting the metabolism. Exercise raises metabolism, right? Yes, but remember that your Physical Activity Level (our old "PAL" from chapter 3) does not make up for the decrease in the Resting Metabolic Rate, because they are different components of metabolism. You may raise your PAL metabolism to a degree, but that RMR, which is so hard to speed back up, will take a hit that is not worth the decrease in calories. You remember the Resting Metabolic Rate: it makes up the largest piece of your calorie burning capacity by doing all of your body's basic maintenance.

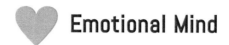 **Emotional Mind**

> Food restrictions create cravings and overeating. Allowing ourselves to eat the foods we want inspires better portion control.

> I can't do anything right. I am a glutton and sugar addict. Maybe a new diet will work.

While our intellectual mind is coming up with a plan for the next diet, our **emotional mind** wants to get on board, but faith is slipping. The emotional mind is remembering all those cravings when calories were low. And instead of recognizing this as biology, we begin to internalize these cravings as personality flaws. We assume that this is because we have been weak and gluttonous. We grab onto fad diet messages that reinforce these beliefs, and then try to follow those diets.

A more appropriate solution to this emotional crisis—and a solution we'll explore later in this book—is to allow ourselves to eat all foods, rather than putting good and bad labels on certain things. This solution actually inspires better portion control, since we do not feel the compulsion to eat it all now because we know we can have it again tomorrow.

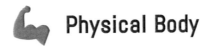 **Physical Body**

> Foods high in fat and sugar have a high satiety value and calorie density. We naturally crave them when our body doesn't have enough calories.

> I am so hungry and need energy. Junk food will have to do since there was no breakfast again today.

On this new diet, as the dieter attempts to manipulate calories again through food restrictions and increased exercise, the **physical body** gets desperate. Not only does the food intake not meet the needs, but there is another source of calorie expenditure as well. Let's take note of yet another precaution the body will take.

Physical Precaution 2: Your body will make you crave high-fat and high-sugar foods! But why? The answer is not that you are a glutton and addicted to sugar, as our intellectual mind and emotional mind (which has been beaten down) would have us believe. These cravings occur because our body wants these foods in order to get calories and feel satisfied. High-fat and high-sugar foods are naturally high in calories and also have an awesome satiety factor. Our body knows that when we eat foods with fat in them, the fat slows the rate at which our stomach empties, keeping us satisfied longer. Our body also recognizes a high-fat food as calorie dense almost immediately, so we feel settled more quickly and can take the meal slowly and steadily. And sugar makes things taste good! Our body recognizes this and knows that we will eat more of it because it tastes good, and more is better because the body does not know when it will get a square meal again. It has no ability to plan ahead because we are acting so unpredictably all the time, and therefore it stores up every single thing that goes down the hatch.

At this point in the cycle, the dieter gets very discouraged. Not only do the food restrictions become harder to maintain, but this newer diet attempt does not yield the same amount of weight loss that the previous diet did. So, at some point, the frustrated dieter is likely to try it all again.

Cycle 3

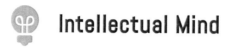

Intellectual Mind

Researching different diets and hyper-focused on physiology claims. Cutting out breakfast to 'save' calories (TEF) or eliminating food groups.

This doesn't make sense, I did it before. I must be more diligent; maybe I'm eating the wrong foods.

Getting ready to embark on yet another diet, the **intellectual mind** now works overtime to try to figure out a solution. We cannot understand why we can't lose weight like we did before. We are searching our brains for logical answers and telling ourselves we just need to be even more diligent. We are researching different diets, seizing onto any diet that seems to have had promising results for our friends. We might take more extreme measures this time, eliminating entire food groups in the belief that we must somehow be allergic or intolerant to those foods. We might cut out breakfast to save calories since we're not hungry in the morning anyway.

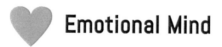

Emotional Mind

Guilt when eating "bad" foods. Cope by mindless eating, which results in overeating without realizing it.

Eating donut just this once...going to have a few since I'll never eat it again. Distractions dull guilt.

While the intellectual mind is problem-solving again, the **emotional mind** hits an all-time low. Guilt sets in, but the mind can't see that the guilt becomes the new underlying reason for overeating.

The internal conversation at this point of the Dieting Trifecta goes something like this: "I really would love to eat one of those doughnuts; they look so yummy. Of course I can't eat doughnuts; they are such a bad food. Well, I've already cheated today anyway, so I'll go ahead and have one, and then get back on track tomorrow. This doughnut is amazing, and after tomorrow I will never let myself have one again because I will begin eating healthy forever. So I ought to go ahead and have a few now." If it's only once in a while that we have an excess of doughnuts or any other high-calorie food (and excess depends on each individual and his or her personal level of fullness), then our body is usually able to make up for the increased calories without gaining weight. Think about that stuffed feeling after a special holiday meal that happens once or twice a year; that is part of normal eating (see Ellyn Satter's "Definition of Normal Eating" in chapter 8). However, when we set up so many constraints around the foods we eat, the Last Supper style of eating becomes more frequent and conducive to weight and health problems.

For many people, the guilt from the emotional mind reaches a breaking point by now. When we believe messages about good and bad foods, constantly trying to avoid what we like while cutting calories—all while also trying to live our lives—something has to give. And we do have to eat, contrary to what diets tell us. So we cope by mindless eating. We eat mindlessly when we eat while distracting ourselves (watching television, reading, talking on the phone). We eat whatever is in front of us, not recognizing the point at which we feel full and satisfied. When this happens only every once in a while, our body is able to make adjustments and return to normal eating. However, when this happens repeatedly, we will gain weight. For constant dieters, distracted eating often becomes a regular occurrence. Here is where we see the paradox: the person trying the hardest to diet and resist food is also the person gaining weight. Yet sadly the eating is never an enjoyable experience. The dieter doesn't get the consolation of telling him- or herself, "Yeah, but didn't we have some amazing meals to show for it." Mindless eating is fraught with guilt, self-loathing, and often no appreciation of taste as favorite foods go down the hatch.

Overweight people often also deal with social discrimination and judgments from others who label them as gluttonous, inactive, and neglectful of their health. Their entire identity can become about their weight, especially when others are talking about and judging them. This creates yet another dynamic in the Dieting Trifecta that can contribute to emotional eating and other coping mechanisms.

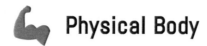

Physical Body

> Body quickly recognizes any calorie deficit and breaks down valuable muscle mass for energy.

> Uh oh, not enough food again. Slow down operations, and break down the easy energy.

Now the **physical body** alternates between being exposed to extremely strict restrictions and bouts of significant overeating. The body reacts swiftly to the calorie deficits and breaks down muscle mass for needed calories. Unfortunately, the added calories during the binge do not re-create the lost muscle.

Physical Precaution Three: Your body has yet another trick up its sleeve: you do not eat enough food throughout the day, so every time the body needs calories to do its work it will break down the muscles that you have worked so hard to build. Muscle is quick energy for the body, no matter how hard it was to earn. Muscle is also very metabolically active, which means the muscle you have is helping you burn more calories and for longer periods of time. It is the last thing you want your body using for the energy it needs to blink and make tears—which you're likely to have a lot of at this point!

And the Cycle Continues

I have noticed an interesting phenomenon in my years of speaking with chronic dieters, counseling them, and reviewing their histories: with each successive diet the dieter embarks on, the length of time that he or she is able to adhere to the diet restrictions becomes shorter and shorter. Finally, simply the idea of beginning a diet is enough to create an episode of Last Supper–style eating with all the guilt and self-loathing that follows.

In order to break the vicious cycle of dieting and escape the Dieting Trifecta, we have to respect and acknowledge the ways that our body, mind, and intellect are in constant interaction with each other. Our nutritional health has a whole lot of systems at play, as this long, complicated chapter illustrates. As we have seen, our body is one big system made up of intricately interacting smaller systems, and no part works in isolation of the other.

Humans are not simple creatures, and, through our higher-order thinking skills, we've managed to make eating—something basic to human survival—a complicated endeavor. Eating can be simple, though, and moving forward we are going to examine the solutions for either getting out of this Dieting Trifecta or not getting sucked into it in the first place. We will look at the bigger picture of eating and explore new perspectives and approaches that allow us to Ditch the Diet for good. In the second half of this book, we will cover some important groundwork and lay a foundation that healthy habits and nutrition can stand on forever.

But, first, just in case you're not quite convinced, let's consider whether there is any such thing as a good diet.

Chapter 5

Is There Any Such Thing as a Good Diet?

Affirmation: I am not a problem to be solved.

IF YOU'VE EVER EMBARKED upon a fad diet, or two, or three, you've probably realized at some point that it was not a good choice. The cabbage soup diet, the grapefruit diet—in hindsight we realize how ridiculous diets like those are. So, after trying a few quick fixes, many dieters then decide it is time to take a different approach. Often, while such a new approach may be less extreme or faddish, it may still fall into the category of a diet—and, therefore, prove equally detrimental and ineffective.

Even diets that seem moderate can still keep you mired in the Dieting Trifecta with the 97 percent of the dieters that end up there. Even though you might receive nutrition education with these diets—about fiber and fat, the importance of fruits and vegetables, and more, maybe even taught by a registered dietitian—one of the big problems with dieting is the mindset that revolves around it. A diet is an all-or-nothing endeavor in which a person is either on the diet and trying to eat according to its strict regimens, or in between diets and eating pleasurably while ignoring food rules and healthy options. As we saw in chapter 2, "The Evolution of a Dieter," when a dieter experiences a little success, they are more likely to subscribe again to the idea that "I'll do better next time and the next diet will work." That mindset causes dieters to stay caught in the Dieting Trifecta, trying one diet after another. Therefore, where someone is in this dieting continuum is a strong predictor for how they handle diet and nutrition information. In the coming chapters we will discuss the vital importance of knowing *how* to eat before moving on to *what* to eat.

Can Your Diet Work?

My initial meetings with clients include a dialogue about their diet history, and they typically start by sharing with me the diets that "worked" for them. "I did Weight Watchers," I often hear, "and it worked for me. I lost 20 pounds." Then I have to explain the glaring paradox of this statement: a diet has "worked" for you only if you are still 20 pounds lighter. If, however, you have gained that weight back, then we need to address the definition of "worked." When dieters say that a diet "worked," they usually mean that it allowed them to take some pounds off for a time. As a nutritionist, I would say a plan "works" only if it keeps the pounds off long-term. If someone eventually gains back the weight they lost, then the fault lies primarily with the act of dieting itself, and some of the concepts that are inherent in diets. Unfortunately, we often tell ourselves the fault is our own, and both the diet plan and society work to corroborate that. We tell ourselves that if we do better next time, we can keep the weight off permanently.

Diets promise results because that is what we want from them. And for a diet program to acquire and retain customers, it needs to deliver results in a timely manner or it loses customers to another company with another program. For this reason, most diets promise rapid weight loss, achieved through plans that are very low in calories. A low calorie count is the common thread; it's the way that low calorie count is framed that determines the difference from one diet to another. And as we learned in chapters 3 and 4, drastic changes and excessive calorie restrictions are not an effective way to elicit permanent weight loss because of their detrimental effect on metabolism and emotional defense mechanisms.

Even when we look at what seems to be a moderate and well-rounded diet, it can still backfire. If programs like Weight Watchers or the Diabetic Meal Plan system worked well for most people, then there would be no need for this discussion. Unfortunately, "results are not typical," as the disclaimer at the bottom of every weight-loss program ad confirms.

Why don't diets work, especially long-term? First, most diets—even nutritionally varied ones—suggest a calorie level that is too low, which leads to hunger, metabolism shifts, and all the negative outcomes that go along with those. Second, once someone has gone on very low calorie diets, then their actual calorie needs moving forward change due to metabolic shifts, rendering standard formulas inaccurate and difficult to predict. Third, all diets begin with altering food intake and focusing on food selection, without addressing the concept of eating competence. As we will learn together in the second part of this book, it's necessary to become a more competent eater before moving on to food selection and eating nutritionally.

Being a competent eater includes a flexibility with eating that comes with trusting yourself. There are many factors through life that can influence our ability to listen to our body (food insecurity/poverty, food restrictions, negative narratives about us), and those begin laying the foundation for believing the messages diets give us. Diets tell us that we cannot be trusted to eat healthily on our own and must follow the diet's strict rules. And the more diets that we engage in, the more heartily we believe and internalize that message. Here is an example of the very nuanced thought processes that can go along with a calorie restriction. Let's say you are working full-time and are on a 1,200-calorie diet. You are watching what you eat and you have your meals figured out. One day at the office, between breakfast and lunch, you find that you're still hungry. You resist the urge to eat, telling yourself that you definitely should not be hungry because you already had a healthy breakfast (yogurt and fruit), and certainly you can wait until lunch. You convince yourself that is what a non-gluttonous person would do. And so you wait. That waiting process involves a lot of self-talk and thinking about food, and by the time lunch arrives, you are starving and the salad you planned is not ringing your bell; but you eat it anyway, reminding yourself that this is how you should be eating, so you must get used to it. Once you get home from work, it is even harder to resist raiding the pantry and scarfing down some snacks, and you are thinking about and craving everything on the "naughty" list.

You resist, though you remain preoccupied with thoughts of food. This goes on through dinner and until bedtime: eating scarcely yet thinking about everything you wish you could eat. It's all worth it, because at the end of the day you can log your calories and see that you hit your intake goal on the mark. Let's consider that this cycle repeats for a few days in a row. Now, you come to a day that you are not all that hungry for some reason. Your breakfast satisfies you until lunch, and you have a smaller than normal lunch which fills you up nicely. After lunch, co-workers offer you a cupcake to celebrate a colleague's birthday. Because of your small lunch, you actually have enough allotted calories/points to eat it. Yet you are not actually hungry for the cupcake for some reason. Your body is trying to tell you that you have eaten the amount of calories that it needs today, just as earlier in the week it was trying to tell you that it needed more calories. Only this time, your emotional mind remembers how terrible it felt to go around hungry, thinking about food all day and wishing for a cupcake. Now that the cupcake is totally earned, there is no way you will pass it up, whether you actually want it or not.

The above scenario will have variations, of course, yet the take-home message stays the same: listening to your body and being flexible with your food choices are essential for making changes that will last a lifetime. The physical cues you receive and the choices they lead you to make will look different for different individuals. It won't be easy to quantify. If that statement makes you uncomfortable, then you may have some work to do in overcoming a common ailment once put into words by Gloria Steinem. She was discussing another topic, but she described a group trying to get over their "addiction to certainty." That idea has resonated with me in my work ever since, especially as I help clients heal from a lifetime of following diets. A diet is difficult to reject when the seller promises "certain" weight loss, along with specific rules to achieve it. We all like to have answers, and we will buy into things if they come with a sense of certainty. A specific meal plan with prescribed calories may give us the certainty we crave, yet it does not always give us the flexibility to listen to our body's cues or to enjoy food. So, aside from the low calorie level which leads to hunger, cravings, and a diminished metabolism, the strict guidelines may not be the answer for someone with a history of chronic diet attempts.

Common Fad Diets

In order to help us spot the pitfalls of dieting, let's look at a few common diets, their premises, and their plans for creating a calorie deficit. A couple have been around for some time, yet continue to get traction here and there, and others are fairly new.

Diet: The Atkins diet

Premise/Rules: No carbs, just protein and fat

How it creates a calorie deficit: Fat and protein slow the rate that the stomach empties, making us feel full longer; and the diet also eliminates 50 to 75 percent of the foods we typically eat.

Diet: South Beach

Premise/Rules: No foods that are "white"

How it creates a calorie deficit: This is a cute way of eliminating carbs again, keeping just high-protein, high-fat foods, but it also eliminates a high percentage of our typical food supply.

Diet: Paleo

Premise/Rules: No foods derived from agriculture, including all cereals and grains as well as dairy

How it creates a calorie deficit: Only meat and vegetables remain as options, so it eliminates 75 percent of our calorie sources.

Diet: The Whole 30

Premise/Rules: Similar to Paleo, no grains or dairy, but only for 30 days as a way to "detox"

How it creates a calorie deficit: This plan eliminates multiple food groups.

All of these fad diets essentially prescribe the same plan: eliminate entire food groups as a way to eliminate calories. There is nothing sexy, magical, or healthy about any of them. In fact, they are valuing weight loss over health. At what point does the benefit of weight loss outweigh the risks and potential for adverse health effects? The answer to that question is highly contested, partly because it is not the same for everyone. I postulate that if you are losing weight quickly, by any of the aforementioned methods, there is a good chance the benefit of weight loss does not outweigh the risks. We have already identified some of the physical and psychological risks of diets. Include with that the fact that the above diets are *only* creating weight loss. They are not providing the variety of foods necessary for a well-rounded diet that is sustainable and crucial for lifelong health.

The Pros and Cons of Diets

When I was growing up and trying to make a decision about something, my mom would always encourage me to make a list of the pros and cons surrounding the issue. This may be a simple concept, yet most of the time I find it to be an effective way to both illustrate and quantify a problem. Getting the thoughts out of my head and onto paper gives me a certain clarity about an issue, whether big or small.

In that same tradition, I have made a list of the pros and cons that accompany dieting. You might consider making your own list or adding to mine below. Note that the list provided here has more than twice as many negatives as positives. See if your own list proves the same.

THE PROS:
- o Diets give us a structured plan to follow with definitive answers. And those answers affirm our success as long as we follow the plan.
- o Some diets provide good nutrition education. They may teach how to read food labels; the nutritional value of fiber, fruits, and whole grains; how to determine serving sizes; what constitutes a lean meat choice; and the like.

THE CONS:
- o It is usually next to impossible to follow every rule of the plan. And when we can't follow the plan, we question our own self-worth. Yet we often go back and pay the diet program even more money as we give it yet another try, and feel even further demoralized.
- o Too much nutrition education all at once is overwhelming. Information needs to be parceled into manageable chunks so that we can actually assimilate it, act on it, and work with it long enough to form some truly lasting habits.
- o A lot of nutrition information and advice offered by fad diets is not credible or evidence-based, and is promoted with anecdotal testimonials. It can be difficult to decipher between the two, especially when diet programs have charismatic and convincing figureheads leading the charge.
- o Any prescribed calorie amount is an educated guess. Most plans come with formulas and specific calorie restrictions. Yet we are all unique with many varying biological factors, so gauging true calorie requirements with a simple formula is an estimate.
- o When we try to stick to a diet, not only will our thoughts be preoccupied with food, but we also stop listening to what our body truly wants and needs. We think we want junk food mostly because we have told ourselves that we can't have it—not to mention we are also hungry.
- o Diets perpetuate a good food/bad food mentality. Thinking about foods as good or bad tends to put eating at the forefront of the mind all the time. A healthier mindset has food at the periphery, taking up some of our time and attention but leaving room for all the other important aspects of our lives.
- o Our body needs only a certain amount of calories each day. When we binge on some days and then fast on others (as is the premise of some diet plans, and tends to happen when a person is dieting anyway), then on the "binge days" the excess calories will be stored as fat, no matter what the source of the calories is, and on the "fasting days" your body is deprived of the calories that it needs and will break down muscle to use for energy.

I hope you're beginning to see all the reasons you should Ditch the Diet once and for all. As we continue through the rest of this book, we will explore ways to address our health concerns that are not centered on diets. We will dig deep into some nutrition concepts, decipher between fact and fiction, and learn how to eat and live more healthfully. The next few chapters focus on real solutions you can turn into lifelong eating practices, including how to eat mindfully, allowing yourself to eat, creating lasting habits, eating nutritionally, and maintaining your physical and psychological health.

Chapter 6
Are You Ready for Solutions?

Affirmation: I can do hard things.

WHENEVER I READ BOOKS that outline a problem, at a certain point I find myself saying, "Yes, I get it, I'm on board. Tell me what the solution is!" So, now that we fully understand the problem of diets, it's time to get on with it. Given the complicated nature of dieting—our bodies, biology, psychology, personal lifestyles, genetics, and more—it is important to recognize that there is no one-size-fits-all solution. However, there are some simple truths that are absolutely beneficial for everyone; with them, we'll offer ways to undo some of the damage already done for those recovering from a lifetime of dieting and ways to prevent future damage for those who have never dieted before.

The solutions I outline here and expand upon in the following chapters represent a journey. Together, we will explore ways to move forward out of a dieting mentality and establish a healthy lifestyle through new habits and a refreshed mindset. These solutions are the meat that you have been waiting for, and they have the cerebral-, action-, and plan-oriented answers you desire, as well as some more nuanced ideas that will have you digging deep. This said, you may find some advice less groundbreaking than you hoped for, yet I encourage you to press on. The real answers to health and longevity are much less dramatic than all the quick-fix miraculous cures splashed across the Internet. Those so-called cures create short-lived buzz with a high price tag for consumers. You may think the solutions I outline are pretty moderate, and sometimes bordering on mundane, but they are absolutely doable and effective.

If we could prevent weight gain and lose weight with "the right diet," then our culture would have hit on that diet by now. Our obsessions with dieting—good foods, bad foods, losing weight, and the like—have been increasingly expansive and inundating over the past 30 years. And yet these obsessions have not resulted in a healthier, fitter, or slimmer society. Something has to change. We must simplify. As much as we want to treat nutrition as scientifically as we do brain surgery, that is not always helpful. We have to combine evidence-based physical and biological research with intuition, personal stories, and well-established psychological and behavioral sciences studies.

Now that we've Ditched the Diet, let's get started with real solutions. If you're a list lover, you'll appreciate this overview of the solutions to be discussed in the remainder of the book. Each of these topics will be covered in detail in the chapters that follow. Our main five solutions are encompassed in the Pyramid to Healthy Eating pictured on the next page.

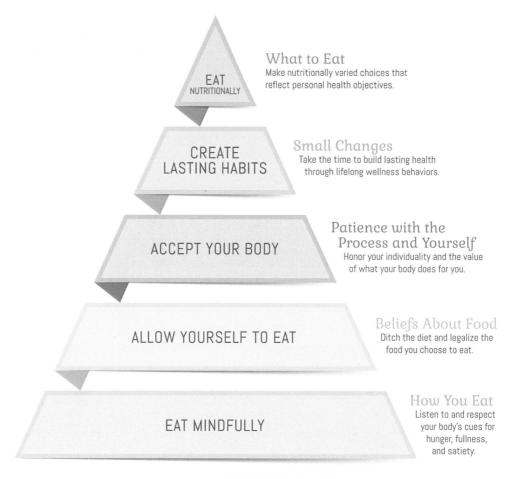

EAT
NUTRITIONALLY

What to Eat
Make nutritionally varied choices that
reflect personal health objectives.

CREATE
LASTING HABITS

Small Changes
Take the time to build lasting health
through lifelong wellness behaviors.

ACCEPT YOUR BODY

**Patience with the
Process and Yourself**
Honor your individuality and the value
of what your body does for you.

ALLOW YOURSELF TO EAT

Beliefs About Food
Ditch the diet and legalize the
food you choose to eat.

EAT MINDFULLY

How You Eat
Listen to and respect
your body's cues for
hunger, fullness,
and satiety.

© 2017 Triple Braided, LLC

The base of this Pyramid to Healthy Eating comprises the foundational concepts that must be mastered before moving to the upper levels. If we skip the steps at the base of the pyramid, then all of our newfound nutrition changes don't have anything to stand on, and eventually end up crumbling. When it comes to nutrition, most people's inclination is to start with *what* to eat, because food choices by themselves are concrete and straightforward. But my Pyramid to Healthy Eating shows that we should first work through some crucial abstract concepts: how you eat, your beliefs about food, and the need for patience with the process and yourself. These steps are about psychologically setting yourself up for success in making healthy nutrition changes. By beginning here, we cover the core elements that ultimately enable us to make good eating choices for life. My hope, as you progress through each of these chapters, is that you will understand how this foundation is essential to your ability to create lasting habits and eat nutritionally. You will also find at the end of each chapter a "Putting It into Practice" worksheet which you can use to track your progress. Here is an overview of what you will learn in each chapter to come.

Chapter 7
EAT MINDFULLY

What exactly does eating mindfully mean? This concept is the base of the Pyramid to Healthy Eating, and while it may feel like a step we are tempted to skip over, it is actually foundational for managing food intake. To explain mindful eating and how we will employ it on our journey, I use the Hunger Dial to teach you about the stages of hunger, satiety, and fullness. The Hunger Dial takes us back to basics with first looking at *how* you eat before overhauling *what* you eat. You have to learn to listen to your body and pay attention to your body's cues while you eat. That can be hard depending upon how much of an intuitive eater you are to begin with. In this chapter we will explore this nuanced idea, and discuss ways to practice it and make it a part of your life.

Chapter 8
ALLOW YOURSELF TO EAT

This chapter may seem to be about *what* we eat, but it is still focused on *how* we eat—or, more specifically, *how we feel* about what we eat. Be flexible, intuitive, and realistic when it comes to food. In other words, you are allowed to eat foods that are not healthy; in fact, you have permission to eat whatever you choose. By taking away the strict dos and don'ts and listening to your body while you eat, you become in tune with your body and recognize its needs and wants with more precision. Amazingly enough, this is a key factor in regulating portions. I want you to liberalize the food choices in your life now in order to help you make more well-rounded nutrition choices that you can feel good about later. You may find that there are some emotions that crop up as you allow yourself to eat that also need to be addressed. That is a good thing, because recognizing the source of your food feelings will give you the opportunity to work on the root of the problem. When we skip straight to food selection first, we set ourselves up for future setbacks before we have even begun.

Chapter 9
ACCEPT YOUR BODY

It's time to talk about our bodies, and the large role that body dissatisfaction plays in our eating and overall health. We need to dispel some common misconceptions about the role of weight in our health, and the parameters that are defining overweight. The pressure and desire to lose weight are so strong that the accompanying emotions often overpower our decision-making faculties. It's hard to accept our bodies, especially when society tells us not to. But this chapter is about learning to feel more at ease with yourself and being patient with yourself and the process of regaining your health. Body acceptance is an essential step toward continuing down the path of physical and mental health and truly being able to eat nutritionally.

Chapter 10
CREATE LASTING HABITS

In this chapter we look at the role of establishing habits in our life. I'll show you how good habits are an important part of treating your body well, plus offer some tips on creating new habits. Creating lasting habits will be the key to making sustainable changes, especially as we learn more about selecting foods and eating nutritionally.

Chapter 11
EAT NUTRITIONALLY

Once we have mastered the skills involved in how to eat and how to think about our bodies and our health, then we can really dive into what to eat. We will be prepared to tackle some nutrition goals without the likelihood of falling back into old patterns and ending up in the Dieting Trifecta. In this chapter, I'll encourage you to enjoy a large variety of foods, and I'll give you some accurate information about foods and their nutritional value. You will learn how to incorporate and enjoy all foods while maintaining a healthy, nutritionally diverse eating style.

Bonus Chapter
BUILD IN EXERCISE

Although exercise is not a part of our pyramid, it certainly is crucial for overall health and well-being. Building up to a goal of daily physical activity is absolutely essential. Our body needs cardiovascular exercise, strength training, stretching, proper breathing, and a regular routine in order to put all the pieces of wellness and nutrition together. In this bonus chapter, I explain how your exercise routine will help your health goals fall into place much more seamlessly. We will look at types of exercise and consider how to create an exercise plan that you commit to and maintain, even with an already full life.

Bonus Chapter
DON'T FORGET YOUR PSYCHOLOGICAL HEALTH
by Kathy L. Sieja, MA, LPC retired

In this final bonus chapter, you will hear from a lifelong family therapist (who happens to be my mother). She describes what she has identified as the six primary aspects of a psychologically healthy person: staying active, sleeping, journaling, attending to your spirituality, socializing, and feeding your brain. You will see how topics from previous chapters come together with some additional concepts to emphasize the importance of our "whole" selves. Each one of us is a big mural made up of many intricate pieces—all of them essential to who we are, how we feel, and how we live.

Chapter 7
Eat Mindfully

Affirmation: My body is wise and my intuition is strong.

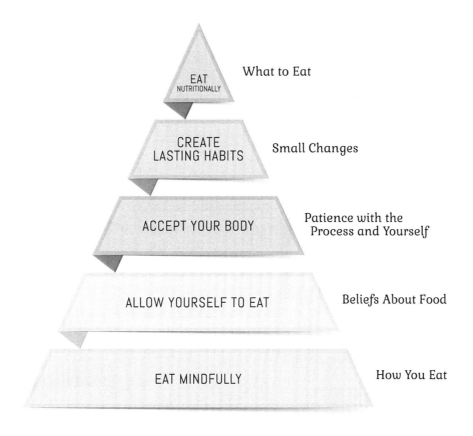

THE HUMAN BODY is brilliant! It provides us a lot of the information we need for optimal performance and health, information we could not possibly learn from reading or researching. Yet we consistently attempt to outsmart our bodies when it comes to eating. If we ever hope to reach the pinnacle of eating nutritionally at the top of the pyramid, we must master one very important foundational skill: eating mindfully.

Let's consider the example of babies. Babies tell us when they are hungry, and likewise they let us know when they are satisfied. As any parent knows, feeding a baby is not a science, as much as we would like it to be. Every child is different, with their own unique eating patterns. I nursed each of my babies, and I was awestruck at how perfectly they demonstrated the concept of internally regulated eating. As a mother nurses, she never knows exactly how much the baby is eating, but she follows the baby's lead and lets that child tell her when it has had had enough, which any infant will do in no uncertain terms. You can't make a baby stay latched on to eat; by the same token, it's pretty impossible to ignore a hungry infant. Sure, many well-meaning parents may attempt to get a baby to eat the "proper" amount; however such efforts may begin to teach children that their own internals cues for hunger/satiety are incorrect and should be ignored. These internal cues are the foundation of this chapter, and by learning to recognize them you will set your body up for eventual success in making nutritionally rich and varied choices.

Listen to your body and be attentive while you eat. This will allow you to recognize your own stages of hunger and satiety. Eat to satisfaction most of the time, and trust your body, because it will help you regulate your eating. When you don't remain aware while you eat, or when you keep yourself distracted while you eat, then you miss your body's cues and risk going straight from hungry to stuffed, without observing the stages in between. Not only can this result in weight gain, but you will also miss out on the opportunity to enjoy your food. When you pay attention during a meal, you will notice when you are pleasantly full, satisfied, and finally finished eating.

Many times, chronic dieters eat in a distracted state because they feel guilty about what they are eating. Inattentive eating is a mechanism for letting ourselves eat something we love without having to think about it and feel guilty. Therefore, part of the mindful eating process means giving yourself permission to eat—even doughnuts or cheeseburgers (more on this in the next chapter, "Allow Yourself to Eat"). When you eat mindfully, your body will tell you when it is done, regardless of what the food is.

To begin to understand mindful eating, let's consider what we are being mindful about. A good place to start is understanding hunger and satiety, and some general physical stages that we go through when eating. Hunger and satiety can be perceived as vague sensations to some, entirely elusive to others, and subjective to many. Unfortunately, there is no scale or thermometer that measures them for us, and they can differ from one day to the next. To help capture some of the nuances involved and teach you some of the cues to watch for, I developed an illustration called the Hunger Dial. On the following page, you can view the Hunger Dial, and in the remainder of this chapter, you can learn how to use it as a tool to help you eat more mindfully.

When we eat mindfully, listening to our body's cues as we eat, we can begin to recognize the stages shown on the Hunger Dial as we experience them. These stages may be more or less recognizable to you depending upon what degree of an intuitive eater you are. People who have struggled with their weight and dieted for extended periods of time may have more difficulty pinpointing the nuances of mindful eating in the beginning. However, with practice and time, you'll start to pick up on your body's cues, and you'll be able to avoid the sort of unconscious eating that takes you from hungry to uncomfortably stuffed, with no awareness of the several stages in between. Instead, you'll learn how mindful eating can let you feed your hunger, enjoy your food, and stop when you feel content and pleasantly satisfied.

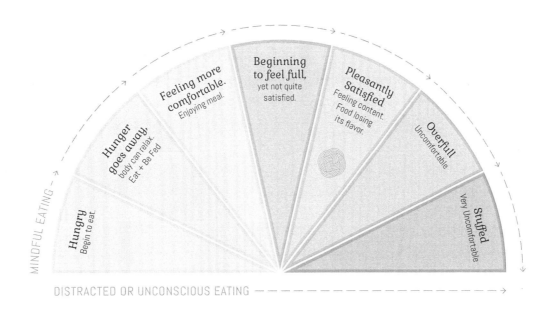

The Hunger Dial

MINDFUL EATING

Look at the Hunger Dial above and notice the dotted line that gently curves over the top of the dial. The best way to begin to understand mindful eating is to trace that dotted line, beginning on the left-hand side with the section titled "Hungry" and moving through each stage until we arrive at the final section on the right titled "Stuffed." Follow along as we learn about the stages of mindful eating.

Hungry

With the Hunger Dial as our guide, let's start with the very first stage of eating: **hungry**. This is the stage we find ourselves in as we sit down to eat a meal. Ideally, we will be hungry, although not too hungry; being too hungry makes it difficult to eat in a mindful manner, since our primordial instincts will kick in to get us fed, which usually leads to speed eating. Therefore, we want to feel ready to eat, but not at the point of raging hunger. We should sit down at the table hungry, and then begin to eat.

Hunger Goes Away

If we are staying mindful as we eat, we may notice that it takes only a few bites before the feeling of **hunger goes away**, as depicted by the second segment on the Hunger Dial. Now the body recognizes that it is being fed, and it begins to settle down. Common confusion at this point arises when the dieter mistakes "hunger going away" for the point at which they should stop eating. This is not the case! At this stage, the body is giving us the opportunity to slow down, chew our food well, and recognize what it tastes like—all contributing to overall nourishment. If we stop eating at this point, which happens sometimes (when we are interrupted, or have only enough time for a few bites, or have limited food available to us), we will find that we feel hungry again in less than an hour or so.

It is important to pause and consider the dieter's experience of this stage, and the emotional consequences it can have. If dieters misconstrue this cue of lessening hunger as a cue for being satisfied or the point at which they should stop eating, then they will be disconcerted and frustrated by the hunger they experience again in 45 minutes. That returning hunger could make them feel innately gluttonous, like an internal flaw they can't control. By extension this can create all sorts of unhealthy ramifications, both emotional and physical. As we have already witnessed, physical hunger paired with emotional distress can make a dangerous combination, because they work together to distort thinking and insist on broad measures to get fed.

Feeling More Comfortable

After those first few bites take hunger away, we arrive at the next stage of **feeling more comfortable** and enjoying the meal. At this point, we are no longer experiencing the gnaw of hunger that originally motivated us to eat; now we can really appreciate the flavors, textures, and individual qualities of the meal. This is a particularly enjoyable stage of a tasty meal because we are able to appreciate the food in a relaxed and mindful state—when we are being attentive, that is.

Beginning to Feel Full

As we continue to eat, we arrive at the phases where things can get dicey. The next two segments of the Hunger Dial are still in the safe zone and are both suitable stopping places to aim for. It depends upon the meal and varying circumstances as to which stage we might choose to stop eating. In the fourth phase, we are **beginning to feel full** yet are not quite satisfied. We experience those initial cues that indicate we may have had enough to eat. At this point, depending on the meal, the food may still be tasting good to us or not, which in turn affects how satisfied we feel. Sometimes when you are eating a ho-hum meal that doesn't particularly ring your bell, you start to feel pretty satisfied at the same time you begin to feel those initial fullness cues. This, then, tells you to end the meal. If you're at a restaurant, ask for a to-go box; when you're eating at home, empty your leftovers into the garbage or place them in a container for later. On the other hand, if you are not feeling satisfied, yet are experiencing those initial fullness cues, you should now slow down and take stock. Put down your fork, chew your food, and assess. As you begin to slow down, are you still not quite satisfied or have you reached the next stage?

Pleasantly Satisfied

When you slow down and take a couple more bites, consider how flavorful those bites are to you now. Now that you have begun to feel the initial cues of fullness, you may notice that the food is beginning to lose its flavor, you are feeling physically content, and you are **pleasantly satisfied**—which means you have reached the next stage on the Hunger Dial. You are not too full, and you can walk away from the meal feeling that you got enough and it tasted great; you are not wishing you had more. This stage is an ideal place to be. And yet it can be a difficult stage to find for yourself. When I discuss the Hunger Dial stages with clients, some immediately recognize them and the feelings associated with them. Others are less sure. They think it sounds logical, yet are not certain they have a recognizable satisfied stopping place. I contend that most of us do. It can take some practice to find it, so here are a few strategies that can help you discern this stage while eating:

- o Minimize distractions.
- o Really focus on tasting your food.
- o Chew your food thoroughly.
- o Slow down while you eat.
- o Take a sip of water after every few bites.
- o Always portion out your food by putting it on a plate, in a bowl, or in a baggie.
- o Assess how satisfied you are before going back for seconds.

Overfull

The next phase in the Hunger Dial comes when we continue to eat, and we pass from pleasantly satisfied to **overfull**. So many factors make it easy to slide from content to uncomfortable: large portion sizes and our natural inclination to finish eating what is in front of us; food prevalence in social circumstances and our desire to partake even when we're satisfied; intermittent access to enough food (as in the case of people living in poverty), which leads to survival-mode overeating when food becomes available; special meals at holidays and occasions when we know we are full but are aware that this special-occasion meal won't come again for a long time. All of these situations may lead us to eat more than we need at a sitting. Even if we are being mindful, we may occasionally make the decision to slide into overfull because of these aforementioned factors. To be clear, we can be a mindful eater and still get to the stage of overfull. The question then becomes, how often do you reach this stage in eating, and is it contributing to excess weight gain? If it happens only intermittently or in response to extreme calorie needs, then your body will generally adapt. However, if you are reaching this stage on a daily basis, despite being able to recognize it as you eat mindfully, then it may be beneficial to develop some techniques for helping yourself stop at the pleasantly satisfied stage. The tips listed above are a good starting strategy.

The examples I've given that tempt us to reach the overfull stage share a common thread. They are all scenarios in which there is increased access to food or food is plentiful at a particular meal. On the surface, having increased access to food may sound like a good problem to have. Yet when you mix food abundance with the ambiguity of not knowing when you will have enough to eat again, then it becomes harder to listen and respond to your own internal stopping place. In other words, even though you may feel full, you might not stop eating because you're not sure when or if you will get to eat this well again. That ambiguity may be due to poverty and compromised access to food, or it may be self-imposed as in the case of a dieter. In the mind of a dieter, that food desert is as chronic and dire as actually having inadequate food resources.

Stuffed

Moving from overfull to the stage of feeling **stuffed** and very uncomfortable is a subtle yet distinguishable transition that most of us can relate to. Feeling stuffed is markedly more uncomfortable than feeling simply overfull, and it takes much longer to recover from. Reaching the stages of overfull and stuffed can happen for similar reasons, and to everyone. It is a normal part of eating to become overfull or stuffed sometimes. Yet reaching this stage of eating frequently could be an important contributor to weight gain. At these stages, our body cannot adjust for the excess in calories and must store them for future use. In terms of calorie balance and weight stabilization, once you are full it is always better to save some of the meal for later than to eat it all now with the plan to fast later to "make up for" the excess calories.

DISTRACTED OR UNCONSCIOUS EATING

We have looked at the seven stages of the Hunger Dial and how we gradually progress through each of these stages if we are eating mindfully. This is a healthy eating process illustrated by the gently curving dotted line that goes from hungry to stuffed. But what happens when we do not eat mindfully? That presents another, negative eating pattern represented by the dotted line that travels straight across the bottom of the dial, directly connecting hungry to stuffed. This pattern occurs with distracted or unconscious eating, the opposite of eating mindfully.

Even within the stages of mindful eating, we have seen places where we can get distracted and thrown off course, thus losing attention to how full or satisfied we have become. We can also begin a meal in a distracted state, which is what we address in this section.

During the process of distracted eating, there is no in between: no tasting, no enjoying, no recognition of getting fuller, no recognition of satisfaction, no feeling … nothing. Nothing until the plate is bare, the meal is over, the bag is empty. Then comes the sensation of being stuffed and very uncomfortably full, along with a rush of unbearable guilt and self-loathing. This dynamic is an unfortunate outcome that arises from a life of repeated dieting. It is the common, frustrating, and heartbreaking consequence that is at the heart of the Dieting Trifecta. The natural, instinctive drive to eat when we are hungry is unparalleled, and the body, mind, and spirit come together in force to get us fed. When we diet, we repeatedly teach ourselves that we are going to be deprived of food at random intervals for extended periods of time; so our body and mind take action to ensure we get food. In part to spare ourselves the guilt that will accompany eating during a diet, the mind shuts off. If the mind thinks, then we might guilt ourselves into not eating, and yet our body is hungry. Thus begins the process of distracted or unconscious eating, which happens when the dieter sits down to eat foods deemed unhealthy/bad/not on the diet/gluttonous. If you are not paying attention, then you can eat it. If you pay attention to what you are doing, then your conscience would say "no"!

Now, getting stuffed and overfull and eating distractedly are not always the results of a dieting history and feelings of guilt surrounding food. Sometimes we just get distracted and don't pay attention, until boom: discomfort! Maybe we get caught up in an engaging conversation or lost in thought, or maybe we have been served a particularly big portion and keep eating to be polite, or perhaps the meal tastes so good and we eat it so fast that our body doesn't have a chance to recognize that we are getting full—until it is too late. There are plenty of reasons for getting overly full. The key is to recognize what is happening with us personally, and to understand that gluttony and lack of willpower may not always be the causes of our overeating.

The moral of this chapter is to relax and trust the process. Our body's appetite will adjust for our nutritional needs even when the reasons cannot be scientifically pinpointed, predicted, or controlled. Now this is not to say that we shouldn't use our higher-order thinking skills! We definitely need to use our mind, too. We are a combination of our intuition, physical body, and brilliant mind. There has to be a good balance between the mind and body.

Given all the choices we have available to us in this modern world, sometimes it can be difficult to tune into what our body needs, or we can be really confused about it. We need solid information to mentally cross-reference with what our body is trying to tell us. Consider this example of how we use our common sense and instincts over and above the rules sometimes. Let's think about children, in particular a sick kid. When a grumpy kid falls asleep in the middle of the day with no other extraneous factors to point to as the reason, many times we discover that they are sick. And isn't it amazing how a sick child may sleep all day and yet still be able to sleep through the night? Our body needs more sleep when we are sick, and even though this extra rest doesn't fit with typical sleep patterns, we don't question its necessity for healing. We trust that the body knows what it needs.

To take this full circle, there are a multitude of reasons why we may feel hungry or not hungry. And many of those reasons are difficult to pinpoint. It could be related to what we have eaten in the past 24 hours, or the degree of physical activity we engage in, or the temperature outside, or environmental factors we were exposed to, or the distribution of the calories we ate, or, or, or … Sometimes we have to be willing to trust sensations that we cannot always explain.

It may be hard not to bring back the question of serving size, and how much we "should" eat. Remember that you need to work on the manner in which you eat first, recognize your hunger and satisfaction cues, and pay attention to how your food tastes. All of these techniques will help you know how much your body needs or wants at any particular meal. Amounts won't always be the same, because there isn't a tried-and-true formula. But once you ditch the diet and heal your relationship with food, then the rest of your nutritional choices will begin to fall in place. And then we can address the more tangible topics of serving sizes and evidence-based nutrition recommendations.

Ultimately, we are trying to find a balance that is real and manageable within the scope of our own lives. That is nearly impossible to do without being mindful. Slow down, chew your food, and really taste what you are eating. Do this without external distractions. I know it is tempting to multitask; however, you will be more successful in recognizing your body's cues when you are free from distractions, especially when you're first learning how to eat mindfully.

Sometimes we eat out of stress or boredom or because a meal is part of a routine. That might be fine, but if we are being mindful, on occasion we will realize that food isn't what we want in a particular moment. If you need to press the pause button before you eat, consider the following list of "stress breakers." These activities are not intended to trick you out of eating; rather they provide ways for you to take a break and decide if a snack is really your desire right then. If so, go for it. If not, you gave yourself a chance to be mindful and figure it out before unconsciously eating. Bravo!

Stress Breakers:
- o   Go for a walk
- o   Exercise to work off steam
- o   Write a letter to a friend
- o   Jot down thoughts in a journal
- o   Play some favorite music
- o   Water your plants
- o   Work in the garden
- o   Rearrange the furniture
- o   Clean out a closet or drawer
- o   Call a friend
- o   Work on a craft
- o   Take a hot bath
- o   Practice a daily relaxation technique
- o   Sew, build, paint, or fix something
- o   Go to a movie
- o   Play with children
- o   Dance in your room

o Talk about your troubles in the mirror
o See a counselor
o Visit a place of worship
o Meditate
o Write poetry
o Watch an educational show on TV
o Wash your car
o Make a list and set priorities
o Tell someone what you really need
o Get a massage
o Take some quiet time for personal reflection

To recap, our goal with eating mindfully is to help our body negotiate the intricate relationship between getting enough of the food that we want for enjoyment and getting enough of the food we need for health. Teaching ourselves how to eat mindfully is the first step in that negotiation. In order to eat mindfully, we must be aware of the stages of hunger and satiety that the body typically goes through, as well as the ways the process can be derailed. Let the Hunger Dial help you master mindful eating, and I think you will be pleasantly surprised by your ability to learn how to stop eating at a place that is both emotionally and physically satisfying.

Putting It into Practice

On a scale of 1 to 10 where would you rank how mindfully you eat overall, with one being *never* or *can't relate* and 10 being *almost always*?

What are your personal challenges to eating mindfully?

What are your goals for becoming a more mindful eater?

What step can you take today to begin the process?

Chapter 8
Allow Yourself to Eat

Affirmation: My mind is clear and open.

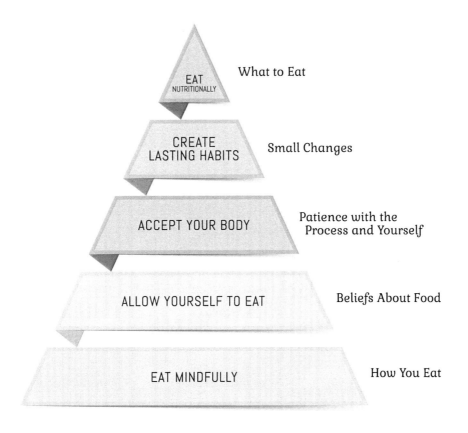

EAT
NUTRITIONALLY — What to Eat

CREATE
LASTING HABITS — Small Changes

ACCEPT YOUR BODY — Patience with the Process and Yourself

ALLOW YOURSELF TO EAT — Beliefs About Food

EAT MINDFULLY — How You Eat

OUR FAMILY HAS had fun lately discussing the different generations—Baby Boomers, Generation X, Millennials, and others coming up on the horizon—and where we all fit in. We know these generations have their own personality traits, largely defined by the early cultural and life experiences of the groups as a whole. And that can even spill over into how each generation relates to food. A prime example is my dad, who has probably had enough of me telling this story (though he knows I do it in love and fondness). As a Baby Boomer and the offspring of the Greatest Generation, my dad was raised "cleaning his plate." My dad always cleans his plate … and the plates of those around him! When someone has gone through the Depression and has known what it feels like not to have enough food, then "wasting" food is not an option. And that is what my dad was firmly taught by his parents. When I was growing up, my father and I had constant battles at mealtime. Not only was I a picky eater as a child, but I was also very internally regulated, so when I was done eating, I was done! Oftentimes that meant a few things left on my plate: one bite of chicken, one piece of broccoli, and one wee pile of rice … oh, and let's not forget the last sip of milk in the bottom of my glass. My dad could not understand how I could leave that small amount on my plate, and it drove him nuts. Today he just rolls his eyes and we have a good laugh about it. But the reason I tell this story is to illustrate the concept of this chapter. My dad would clean his plate regardless of whether he was full or not because he was taught to do that by people who cleaned their plates out of hunger. And his parents, because of their history, were frugal with the amount of food they bought. They didn't have a pantry and refrigerator packed with food, and when his mother prepared a meal, he ate it.

In this chapter we will discuss our beliefs about food, specifically the beliefs related to our access to food and permission to eat it. My grandparent's generation experienced a time of widespread food insecurity that was so impactful that even the next generation learned to feel obligated to eat what they were given. By contrast, when we know that we have plenty of access to food, then there is less reason for us to feel compelled to eat.

As we move to the next level of the Pyramid to Healthy Eating, once we are eating mindfully, now we can allow ourselves to eat and begin to trust ourselves with any and all foods. The goal is to be flexible, intuitive, and realistic with food choices. This means you are also allowed to eat foods that are not healthy; in fact, you have permission to eat whatever you choose. By taking away the strict dos and don'ts and listening to your body while you eat, you become in tune with your body and recognize its needs and wants with more precision. Amazingly enough, this is a key factor in regulating portions. Sometimes a realistic food choice is not the healthiest option, but with the unpredictability of life we must eat what we can sometimes. This is where being flexible and intuitive play a part. Of course, access to solid nutrition resources is important. However, at this point in our journey toward healthy eating, we want to suspend our judgments about how nutritious particular foods are as we work to renew or preserve eating competence.

Whether you are a recovering dieter or someone wanting to make more nutritious choices, you need to be able to internalize and embrace the idea that you can be trusted to eat any food you choose. And you must accept that, most of the time, you will be able to stop eating at a portion size appropriate for you. You need to know that it is acceptable to eat doughnuts as long as you pay attention while you eat and can recognize the stages of the Hunger Dial. Wait … what? This can be a difficult concept and may take a minute for you to wrap your head around my advice. Remember our discussion of the Hunger Dial in chapter 7? One of the reasons the dieter overeats is that they feel guilt and shame when eating "bad" foods. When we choose to eat foods we feel are "bad" for us, we intentionally eat them mindlessly, and that's when we ignore the cues of fullness and satiety that our bodies are giving us. If no foods are completely off-limits, then there is no reason for guilt and shame while eating. And if there is no guilt and shame, then there will be no desire to try and stuff down food without thinking about it. So, to eat a meal mindfully and to be able to find our personal stopping place, we must know that we are allowed to eat the food in the first place.

Now, none of this is cut and dry. Not much having to do with individuals, human nature, food, and emotion is ever cut and dry. Every person's situation is as unique as their body and their life experiences. This stage of allowing yourself to eat is a step in renewing eating competence and it can be a lengthy process. Yet it is foundational to having a healthy relationship with food and should be a primary focus for those recovering from dieting as well as an important food philosophy to be embraced by our whole society.

Food Rules

Why is it so hard to allow ourselves to eat? Part of the problem lies in the current societal conversation surrounding food, dieting, and health. All the strict rules that have developed over the past few decades have backfired. We are heavier, more confused, and less healthy than ever. Our attempts at weight loss and the idea that less weight at any cost will make us healthier have created a cultural eating crisis. Food manufacturers have capitalized on consumers' enormous economic resources, our pleasure-seeking instincts, and our confusion, giving us a wealth of foods that have been engineered and fabricated to meet every possible diet claim while also tasting palatable and being quick, easy, and portable! Many diet claims began as honest labeling that provided ingredient information for people with specific food allergies. However, it has been heightened to a new level. Our culture has gone way beyond health and beyond providing helpful information for those with allergies. Now, all of a sudden we are all allergic—to everything!

Let's take a look at some of the most common claims we see on food packages and in dieting regimens. You'll recognize many of these claims believed by the average consumer to make a food "healthy":

- o Gluten-free
- o Soy-free
- o Dairy-free
- o Wheat-free
- o Sugar-free
- o Low-carb
- o No artificial flavors
- o Dye-free
- o Vegan
- o No GMO
- o Hormone-free
- o Grown without pesticides
- o High-protein

    o   Organic
    o   Paleo
    o   Grain-free

If we eat according to these claims, will we have a healthy diet? Should we follow all of them or pick just a few? How do we decipher what is applicable for us personally? Most of these claims have come about because of heightened awareness surrounding allergies or other health concerns, fad diets, or food production methods. Consider these:

    o   A claim aimed to help certain small groups of people with specific allergies to be able to traverse the world of packaged foods. Example: "Gluten-free" foods intended for people with celiac disease (more on this later).

    o   A claim derived from a fad diet that was popularized to such an extent that the food industry created products to meet the diet's standards or started labeling an already-compliant food with that claim in order to cash in on the fad. Example: "Low-carb" foods as part of a fad diet purely for weight loss, without regard for health (more on this later, too).

    o   A claim intended to alert certain interest or activist groups to a product's compliance with specific environmental or economic standards; food processing, growing or manufacturing practices; religious tenets; or other standards. Example: "Organic" foods as a reaction to concerns with pesticide residues on our food supply.

Some of these claims have merit and can be useful to certain people. But such claims in and of themselves do not make a food a shoe-in for health, an innately better choice, or something that meets the needs of all eaters. Some of these claims actually lead people to make choices that are unhealthy, uncorroborated by research, and may do more harm than good. If you are going to embrace the premise that you are allowed to eat—as I hope you will—it is important to clarify some of these food-restriction claims, although each one on its own could take up scores of books. We can't launch a full-fledged investigation into each, but I'd like to offer an overall conceptual way of thinking about the mass of claims out there.

GLUTEN

Let's start with the example of gluten. Average Americans have by now been so inundated with the phrase "gluten-free" that most probably believe the term is synonymous with a healthy choice. And the majority of us don't even know what gluten is. Gluten is a protein found in wheat, rye, and barley. It gives bread structure due to its properties of elasticity. About 1 percent of the population has celiac disease, which is an allergy to the protein gluten.

    It is difficult to avoid gluten in the typical American diet, since it is found naturally in foods like breads, pasta, crackers, cookies, and cereals. Twenty years ago, before the food industry had made a gluten-free version of so many foods, people with celiac disease had few options. They generally needed to consult with a dietitian about how to find foods that are naturally gluten-free and devise a plan to meet nutrition needs that way. Today the options are much more palatable, as foods of all kinds have undergone manipulations to make them gluten-free and tasty, too.

This is good for the 1 percent of Americans with celiac disease, who need to eliminate all gluten from the diet, and also for individuals with non-celiac gluten sensitivity (NCGS), who find it helpful to limit gluten. For much of the population, however, going gluten-free has become a fad that people follow with the hopes of losing weight or reducing stomach discomfort. In many cases, this is pure overkill, a common case of throwing the baby out with the bathwater. Even for people with NCGS, the elimination of all gluten isn't typically necessary. In cutting out gluten, people are also eliminating a whole lot of important foods and nutrients unnecessarily.

Gluten is found naturally in any food made from flour: breads, pasta, crackers, and the like. In addition to gluten, flour also contains wheat. Most foods that are gluten-free are also wheat-free. Wheat is the carbohydrate component of the flour, while gluten is the protein component. Wheat falls into a group of carbohydrates called oligosaccharides. Other foods that fall into this category include onions, garlic, legumes, and a variety of fruits, nuts, and vegetables—all very beneficial foods, and important for humans' health. One source of their health benefits is also the same reason that they can bother some people's stomachs. They are indigestible fibers (you may have heard them referred to as prebiotics) because humans don't have the enzymes to break them down in the small intestine. Therefore, they travel to the large intestine and become food for the bacteria that live there, the byproduct of which is gas; this is the natural gas that we have. For some people this gas can be bothersome, even painful, causing bloating, diarrhea, and/or constipation.

Do you see where I am going with this science lesson? By uniformly eliminating gluten from the diet, a whole lot of other things are also being eliminated, things that may be the true source of someone's digestive problems, other than the gluten. And if the problem is something else, then eliminating the gluten may eliminate both more and less than is necessary—more of the foods that are not a problem and less of the foods that are! We should also use this logic to reexamine many other foods that get categorically eliminated and falsely accused as the culprit, such as dairy, soy, fruits, peanuts, grains, and more.

Macronutrients: Uses and Abuses

Quick nutrition 101 lesson: in the science of nutrition and metabolism, foods are categorized into macronutrients and micronutrients. Macronutrients are the nutrients consumed by organisms in large quantities that provide energy (calories). The three macronutrients are carbohydrates, protein, and fat. Micronutrients are the nutrients required in trace amounts for normal growth and development that do not provide energy. Micronutrients include vitamins and minerals.

All three macronutrients—carbohydrates, protein, and fat—are essential in large quantities (hence the "macro") for normal growth and development. Through years of research, scientists have determined a general guideline stating approximately what percent of the diet each macronutrient should comprise for optimal functioning and health. In the same way that the three components of metabolism (Resting Metabolic Rate, Physical Activity Level, and Thermic Effect of Feeding) have a range for what percentage they make up of an individual's calorie burn, there is a range for macronutrient distribution as well.

Here are the Acceptable Macronutrient Distribution Ranges (AMDR) set by the Food and Nutrition Board of the Institute of Medicine. These ranges vary a bit more for children between ages 1 and 3:

	Children	Adults
Protein	10–30%	10–35%
Carbohydrates	45–65%	45–65%
Fat	25–35%	20–35%

These ranges can differ depending upon personal health circumstances as well as individual dietary choices. What meets one person's needs may not be perfect for another. However, these ranges provide a helpful framework to work within.

The manipulation of these percentages has become a common fad diet promotion. Over the years, as I've calculated my clients' intakes and looked at their distribution, I often find that the way people instinctively eat and put meals together usually falls within the acceptable ranges. So it's particularly obvious when someone is following a fad diet and turns in a food record intake with unusual ranges. An intuitive diet does not have 10 percent of calories from carbohydrates.

FAT, CARBOHYDRATES, AND PROTEIN

Our body needs fat, carbohydrates, and protein to function optimally. There are minor deviations in the appropriate proportions of each of these macronutrients for different individuals and to meet various needs. Again, we are all made differently. However, the guidelines listed above give us a good indication for how much of each nutrient will contribute to optimal health.

Fat

Just the word "fat" makes people recoil from its palpable negative connotations! Partially for that reason, fat was the first macronutrient to become the focus of fad diets. Come to think of it, fad diets make nutrition a lot like middle school: a food is part of the in-crowd one day, and then on the outs the next. Of the three macronutrients, fat is the most calorie-dense. That means it contains more calories per gram than either carbohydrate or protein—over twice as much, in fact. Therefore, when one is counting calories, you can get the same amount of calories in a cheese cube or a tablespoon of butter as you would in a half cup of rice. When this information was compounded with some correlations between saturated fat, cholesterol, and heart disease, a new fad was born of some scientific trends and nutrition recommendations. When the average American was encouraged to limit their fat as it would help them to lose weight, another correlation arose. Fat in food must equal fat on the body. Thus began the counting of fat grams instead of calories. Fad diets gave people a number of fat grams to stay below in order to lose those unwanted pounds. "Eat whatever you want as long as you have only 20 grams of fat per day." In response, the food industry created all kinds of processed foods that would allow us to eat tasty foods without fat—but with no regard for the calories or sugar. There was an explosion of fat-free cookies, cakes, crackers, even butter and cheese! You name it, you got it "fat-free." Now, considering that fat adds flavor to foods, those fat-free cookies needed something extra to be palatable: a whole lot of sugar. And since fat helps our bodies feel satisfied, when it's missing from the cookies, then we have to eat a lot more to get that content feeling. Then, since carbohydrates empty out of our stomachs the fastest, all those calorie- and sugar-dense cookies leave us feeling hungry again in a short time. But, if the count is all about fat grams, then heck—how about having some more cookies!

Yet fat in the diet does not equal fat on the body, although fat on and in the body is extremely important. For starters, fat helps cushion our organs, contributes to the manufacturing of hormones, is a key element in decreasing inflammation in the body, makes food taste delicious, and can make meals satiating! In chapter 11, we will dig into the nuts and bolts about fat: kinds of fat, additional benefits, and how to find the healthy ones in food.

Carbohydrates

Our bodies utilize carbohydrates as our primary energy source; they are also a natural source of both soluble and insoluble fiber and a plethora of phytochemicals, vitamins, and minerals that work synergistically to provide us with disease-prevention benefits. That means that the fibers, phytochemicals, vitamins, and minerals work better together and when found in their natural food sources (grains, fruits, legumes, vegetables). Therefore when restricting carbohydrates in an attempt to cut calories, valuable nutrients are also being restricted. A common justification by diet enthusiasts is that they are replacing the micronutrients found in those foods with supplements. However, because of the synergistic value, which subsequently is difficult to measure, taking supplements does not replicate the value provided by the natural food source.

How did carbohydrates get such a bad rap anyway, especially considering how beloved they were in the 1980s? Fat had a bad go for a while, and then carbs got caught up in the fray. As with fat, the real culprit is not the carbs. The problem is multifaceted and is ultimately the result of taking pieces of information in isolation rather than within the scope of a broader picture. We have an insufficient understanding of biology, we want a simple answer, and the diet and food industry is willing to provide that answer. That leads us to following a diet lacking necessary macronutrients with all of the dieting ramifications (Dieting Trifecta) that entails.

Strictly limiting carbohydrates will often lead to an initial weight loss. While you have heard this before, and it may sound clichéd, that initial weight loss and the look of more muscle definition are due in fact to water loss. Your skin will look more buoyant and full when carbs are in your diet, because they help you stay hydrated. Restricting carbs may also provide weight loss because we're likewise limiting the variety of foods we eat, which ultimately puts the dieter in a calorie deficit (the true reason for weight loss). Protein and fat slow the rate at which the stomach empties, so if we avoid carbs, then all we have left are protein and fat, foods that help us stay full longer. Great, right? Sure, but this is not a long-term solution, considering we could enjoy the best of taste and health by having all three macronutrients in all our meals.

Protein

Protein is another essential macronutrient, and consuming the proper amount is important, especially if we understand how it is used and eliminated by the body. There is a limit to how much a body can use and process. Protein is used for healing and building, and the amount that individuals require depends on a number of factors: weight, health, and activity level, to name a few. Protein is generally needed in higher-than-average amounts for people who are ill, recovering from surgery or a wound, or extremely physically active. Even for these select groups, the amount of protein that can be utilized by the body is limited. Approximately 25 grams of protein in a sitting is the most that our bodies can synthesize at once. If a person is consuming more than that, the excess is either being used as an alternate energy source or being stored as fat if energy needs have already been met.

Here is an analogy to illustrate this concept: when building a house, there is a specified amount of lumber needed to frame the structure. If lumber is left over after framing, the builder is not going to tack extra lumber onto the existing frame. Instead, it will be stacked and stored in the shed or used for a different project. Similarly, excess protein will not build bigger muscles; the necessary amount will be used to do repairs, and the excess will be repurposed or stored as fat.

It is also important to understand that protein is the only macronutrient that is not a "clean burning fuel." In other words, as protein is metabolized and broken down, it creates byproducts that must be detoxified and eliminated by the body. Our body is specifically equipped to detoxify certain amounts of protein, but a constant stream of mega-doses could have health consequences down the road.

The foods that contain protein also contain other nutrients that are important for overall health, but they do not contain all of them. There is a huge host of nutrients and functions provided by fat and carbohydrates that cannot be replicated by protein. That is also the case with both carbohydrates and fat, which is why all three macronutrients are necessary for optimal health.

Just Tell Me What to Do …

Sometimes having to make decisions is the hardest part of maintaining a well-rounded diet, and that makes a fad diet feel like a relief: no thinking or decisions; just eat exactly what is on the plan and nothing that is not. That can sound easy, appealing, and even energizing. The problem is that, for most people, the easy and energizing phase lasts only a short time, and then the plan becomes cumbersome and boring. And we are hungry.

Let's back up for a moment and pull all these pieces together to look at how we can approach eating. How can we find an approach that allows us to move food out of the center of our lives and place it on the periphery where it belongs? How can we reach a point where thinking about food and nutrition takes up some of our time and attention, yet does not consume our thoughts and emotions? The answer lies in giving ourselves permission to eat. If you have never had eating issues, weight concerns, or early-life pressure to eat a certain way, you may already allow yourself to eat. If this is the case, you want to stay in a place that is psychologically healthy. Either way, it is probably important to make dietary shifts away from eating habits that are not serving our health well. Those shifts can be accomplished in ways that are small, manageable, and contribute to a happy and healthy lifestyle. I admit that it's not always going to be easy or fun to eat healthfully, but it should not be hard and miserable. Eating should roll with your life. Sometimes it goes smoothly and other times it feels completely erratic and out of control. This is normal!

DEFINITION OF NORMAL EATING

Ellyn Satter is a dietitian and family therapist who created the widely applied division of responsibility in feeding as well as the Satter Eating Competence Model. Years ago she created a Definition of Normal Eating that I consider to be foundational in instilling positive attitudes about eating. She succinctly put into words much of what I want to express to everyone about eating.

Normal eating is being able to eat when you are hungry and continue eating until you are satisfied. It is being able to choose food you like and eat it and truly get enough of it—not just stop eating because you think you should. Normal eating is being able to use some moderate restraint on your food selection to get the right food, but not being so restrictive that you miss out on pleasurable foods. Normal eating is giving yourself permission to eat sometimes because you are bored, sad, happy, or just because it feels good. Normal eating is three meals a day, or it is choosing to munch along. It is leaving some cookies on the plate because you know you can have some tomorrow, or it's eating more now because they taste so wonderful when they are fresh. Normal eating is overeating at times, even feeling stuffed and uncomfortable. It is also undereating at times and wishing you had more. Normal eating is trusting your body to make up for your mistakes in eating. Normal eating takes up some of your time and attention, but keeps its place as only one important area of your life. In short, normal eating is flexible. It varies in response to your emotions, your schedule, your hunger, and your proximity to food.

I find this to be a beautiful and liberating definition of what is normal in the realm of eating, and it sets a realistic stage for people as they look at their personal eating patterns. Once we relax some of the rules related to food, it becomes much easier to make the tweaks and adjustments to our nutrition that will ultimately facilitate a healthy lifestyle. In the next few chapters I will explain how to relax the rules you set for yourself and find manageable ways to make eating changes that really matter. In the process, we'll see that all foods can fit intuitively into a healthy lifestyle without intense do-and-don't micromanaging.

For most people, it is unrealistic to assume that because they know what to eat, they are able to stick to those rules. Having good nutrition knowledge—like knowing what foods help prevent diseases, trying to eat a well-rounded diet, and so on—is important. In fact, solid nutrition knowledge is so incredibly important that I advise getting this information from credible nutrition professionals (RDs or RDNs). See appendix A, "Where to Find Good Nutrition Information," for an explanation of credentialing terms and tips on how to find and vet a credible nutrition professional. This is especially important in these days of pseudo-science and sound-bite information overload that is insidious and viral in our lives. Yet, as is the focus of this chapter, we don't want to put the cart before the horse by jumping to the top of the Pyramid to Healthy Eating before we have mastered the bases. To eat mindfully and to allow yourself to eat are big pieces of the foundation that will help prevent a return to the Dieting Trifecta.

Putting It into Practice

How will knowing and understanding some of these facts about food and nutrition help you feel more empowered to allow yourself to eat?

What information in this chapter most resonated with you?

How will you use this knowledge to give yourself permission to eat?

Chapter 9
Accept Your Body

Affirmation: I am strong. I am beautiful. I am enough.

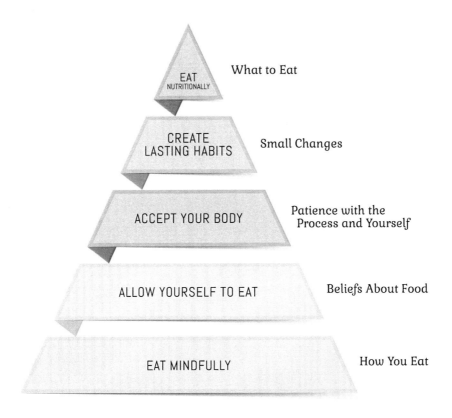

EAT NUTRITIONALLY — What to Eat

CREATE LASTING HABITS — Small Changes

ACCEPT YOUR BODY — Patience with the Process and Yourself

ALLOW YOURSELF TO EAT — Beliefs About Food

EAT MINDFULLY — How You Eat

NO ONE REALLY WANTS to talk about the topic of the body, yet it is something the recovering dieter must consider, not to mention a subject our whole society should address. As we Ditch the Diet and work our way up the Pyramid to Healthy Eating, we won't build habits overnight, so we need to learn to live in our skin while we do the slow and steady work. You may not love your body, but you need to accept and appreciate it. That is a tall order for every one of us, and I recognize the hundreds of objections that you might want to raise in response:

- o   Accepting my body is giving up on being healthy.
- o   Accepting my body means I am okay with the status quo in my life.
- o   I can't accept my body because I hate it.
- o   To be happy I have to get the weight off.

o　This is not my true weight, and I am unwilling to accept it.
o　It would be easier to accept my body if society would also.
o　I don't know how to accept my body as it is now.

Wow, there is so much pain wrapped up in this physical package that holds our precious souls. And so much of that pain stems from societal messages and some common misconceptions. All these thoughts and feelings come from very real places, and it's probably impossible to erase them altogether. Yet, as you do the work to improve your health, I want you to also work toward a new way of thinking about your body. In this chapter, let's see if we can clear up some of the associations we make between life, happiness, and size.

Accepting your body is not akin to renouncing your health. It is a required step on the way to getting healthy. In chapters 7 and 8, I discussed the importance of learning *how* to eat before you can jump into *what* to eat. But there's a crucial component that bolsters those two concepts and processes: body acceptance.

What Constitutes Overweight?

This is an extremely loaded question, and should take into account a multitude of factors. However, our society likes to use a formula to place people in definitive groups. We use tools like BMI (body mass index), the Metropolitan Life height and weight charts, waist to hip ratio, and a host of other formulas to determine whether someone is overweight or not. For some of us, the charts may provide a guideline with some degree of accuracy, while for others the charts can be way off the mark. Our body types are as diverse as our faces, and our bodies change over time. We must also take into consideration the large influence of genetics (as discussed in chapter 3) on our body shape and size—especially as we age. Charts and formulas aside, we all have a weight range and size that we are personally comfortable with and feel is appropriate for us. Again, our preferences can be somewhat accurate, but can also be skewed. It's hard to have an unbiased opinion about weight given the influences of our society and our personal interactions and experiences.

As a dietitian, when I'm working with clients I don't take weight numbers at face value. I'm careful about how I use charts and formulas, and I question each person's perceptions about his/her body. To form a complete picture and plan, I have to know your background and health history and your family's health history and body types. I learn about your lifestyle, activities, sleep patterns, and stress levels. These pieces of information help us determine what kind of weight you're carrying—and, most important, how that relates to your health and longevity.

Weight and Health

Does weight accurately depict health? There is certainly strong evidence to support that it does. The correlation is much stronger in some cases, and with certain weights, than in others.

However, the connection is not as definitive or as cut and dry as some of the rhetoric would have us believe. And the impact of yo-yo dieting and extreme weight fluctuations throughout a lifetime has added a new dimension to the problem. It has made the possibility of weight loss less predictable and less likely. And yo-yo dieting has become its own risk factor because of the negative effect weight fluctuations can have on our health.

To be healthy, does the overweight lifelong dieter have to get back to the weight chart number or size from their young adult years? Is that even a realistic possibility? And is taking off weight at a rapid rate ultimately healthy? Is it going to stay off? The answers to these questions depend upon different factors. The person who has lost and gained weight repeatedly for many years is in a different place physically, metabolically, and emotionally than the person who decides for the first time to make some moderate eating and exercise lifestyle changes through building new habits.

I believe that weight is not the sole predictor of health, and to set weight as the ultimate goal and measure of success is a mistake. In fact, I strongly believe that making weight the be-all and end-all actually makes weight loss less likely. Because an individual weighed a certain amount in the past does not necessarily make that number attainable today. We cannot and should not try to predict what weight will do during a weight-loss attempt. Instead, let's see how changing our focus from body shaming to self-acceptance can set you up for success.

Body Weight and Happiness

It is a pervasive idea that weight loss will produce happiness in our lives. Why is that? Maybe it is comforting to believe that weight loss—something so seemingly objective and straightforward—can improve the way we see the world and live in it. Happiness is an abstract concept, yet a goal that drives practically everything we do. So it makes sense that we look for concrete ways to achieve that abstract feeling. Of course, as this book shows, there is nothing concrete, objective, or easy about weight loss, and it is certainly not straightforward. Yet, in a society teeming with so many negative ideas about weight and body type, it may seem as if having the perfect body would be the obvious way to fit in and feel admired. However, weight loss is almost never the most direct path to happiness. For the past 10 years I have kept this quote by Lao Tzu above my desk as a reminder that happiness is primarily a state of mind: "Be content with what you have; rejoice in the way things are. When you realize there is nothing lacking, the whole world belongs to you."

How to Accept Yourself: The Baby Steps

Let me restate an important point: accepting your body does not mean you should not care about it, and that you should surrender to the idea that your body will never change. I'm not simply telling you to get over it. Acceptance means appreciating yourself and living in your own skin while you do the slow work of creating new sustainable habits in your life. To help you climb up this major step on the Pyramid to Healthy Eating, let's look at some strategies for self-acceptance that will encourage you to change your thought processes in order to serve your ultimate health and nutrition goals.

SIX STRATEGIES FOR SELF-ACCEPTANCE

1. Don't Compare

When we compare ourselves to others, we will always lose. We are not meant to be anyone other than ourselves, with all the unique attributes, gifts, and talents that only we possess. Our human tendency to compare crosses over into every area of our lives, but it is especially tough when it comes to body ideals. Often, we look at someone else's body and imagine that the rest of their life mirrors what we see on the surface: "I know I am a gifted *artist/accountant/ fill-in-the-blank*," we might think, "but if I could have a body like *hers/his* I would be so much more *successful/satisfied/fill-in-the-blank*."

From the outside, we create a picture of what we think another person's life looks like, but we all know that appearance is not reality. And in the same way that losing weight isn't the most direct route to happiness, neither is comparing our body to someone else's a very effective motivator. Nor is it realistic. Instead of comparing your body to another's, appreciate it instead. You can allow yourself to feel envious for a moment, but don't dwell on it. Let it go, and then come up with something that you value about yourself.

2. Change Your Focus

When you focus on aspects of your body, yourself, and your life that you love and are proud of, you employ a powerful tool for positive change. By contrast, shame is a downer, a depressant, and an avenue to anxiety and negative thoughts. It is the opposite of motivating and invigorating, and it almost never inspires positive change. Focusing on the parts of us that we are displeased with probably just sabotages us further. Do you want to go outside for a brisk walk when you feel depressed and sad? I know I don't. When I feel down and am beating myself up about something, all I want to do is sleep to escape the downward spiral of sadness and inadequacy. However, gratitude inspires an entirely different set of thoughts, feelings, emotions, and actions. When we focus on what our body is doing for us and all the ways it allows us to be active and participate in life, then our whole being is lifted and energized. That is the kind of positive energy that moves us forward and gets things done.

In concrete terms, this means you shouldn't fixate on what you don't like right now. For example, don't keep checking out your rear end in the mirror and lamenting about how it used to look 30 pounds ago. Admire your shoulders instead, and how great they look in your new razor-back workout top. Again, I'm not suggesting that we settle for the status quo. But we should strive to live a good and happy life while we take the time to gradually improve our eating and our health. We can choose to focus on our assets. And I know for certain that each and every person has plenty of assets to choose from.

3. Create a Personal Mantra/Affirmation

A mantra can help you shift your mindset both in the moment and over time. Typically a mantra would be a short statement, word, or even sound that can be used to change your focus or zero in on a different thought process.

How might mantras help with body acceptance? It's tricky to come to terms with our bodies and to be appreciative and accepting of the current state of affairs, because life gives us constant reminders and messages that promote the opposite—from mealtimes to mirrors to daily conversations. It is helpful for the brain to have a standard response we can conjure up before we head down the rabbit hole. Shifting your mind from negative to positive is not easy, but it is doable—and we can do hard things.

What kind of mantra should you use? Try something like a mix of a positive affirmation and a personal theme song. You want it to be simple yet personally effective, and you have to be willing to be open-minded. Here are some mantra examples:

- o I am worthy
- o I can choose positive thoughts
- o I surround myself with loving people
- o I am enough
- o I respect the wisdom of my body
- o I am strong
- o I value progress, not perfection
- o I am beautiful right now
- o My body does not determine my self-worth
- o Happiness is beautiful
- o I am thankful for my body and what it can do for me
- o I am capable
- o Strong mind means strong body
- o I can listen to my body
- o I am authentic and uniquely me
- o My eyes reflect the beauty of the world around me
- o I am confident in my decisions
- o I am allowed to take up space
- o My body is mine and mine alone

Because I believe affirmations can make a real impact on the way we think and act, I have included them at the top of each chapter. Take notice of these affirmations throughout the book, and let them guide you as you leave dieting behind and climb the Pyramid to Healthy Eating. Then create a few affirmations of your own.

4. Move Your Body

Let your body show you what it can do! Not only does activity promote the release of endorphins, which make us feel good (serving as our own internal mood enhancers), but activity also inspires all sorts of other positive and productive thought processes. After you start moving, I bet you find that you are amazed, appreciative, and proud of what you can do.

Whether or not our physical activity is actually changing the shape of our bodies, somehow it does change how we see ourselves. You will likely view your body in a more positive light when you recognize and are grateful for its capabilities.

5. Embrace Clothes That Fit You Now

Have you got a closet full of clothes you're saving for the day they'll fit again? If so, that wardrobe is not motivating you. It's actually shaming and discouraging you. You may love that outfit, you may have spent a lot of money on it, and it probably has sentimental value. But believe me when I say, if it no longer fits, it is doing more harm than good hanging there. Your smaller clothes had their day. It is time for you to move on by setting effective, positive goals that will motivate you in the right direction. A tiny talisman in the form of bygone jeans is not that goal. Give them away to a new home and spend a little money on something you love that fits right now!

Part of the process of body acceptance includes buying yourself clothes in your current size that are nice and that you love. Focus on styles, colors, and patterns that accentuate what you like most about yourself: a bright blue shirt that makes your eyes pop, a cute bohemian skirt that shows off your strong calves, bracelets that accentuate your perfectly manicured nails.

6. Build Someone Else Up

Notice the positive qualities in others and tell them. Let the people in your life know the things you appreciate and admire about them. (Now, be careful you don't use this as an opportunity to compare!) Pass out compliments without holding yourself to those particular standards. As we notice and appreciate others, we also give ourselves a message that we are good enough—and even awesome!—just how we are. You may make someone else's day in the process, or set a positive example for a friend.

Take these six self-acceptance strategies in bite-size pieces, and find simple ways to apply them in your life. I would suggest choosing one per week or even one per month, and then read the strategy each day. Be mindful about your intent to work on accepting your body, and employ one strategy with that intent as your focus. Take as much or as little time with each goal as feels right for you. You may find that you want to try only one of the strategies, and that is just fine. You may come back to this book in a few months and find that another strategy speaks to you. Don't ever dismiss the power of proper timing.

In an effort to find happiness through self-acceptance, look at your life from a perspective of abundance, and make a conscious effort to focus each day on a few things you are grateful for. According to Shawn Achor in the book *The Happiness Advantage*, "countless studies have shown that consistently grateful people are more energetic, emotionally intelligent, forgiving, and less likely to be depressed, anxious, or lonely … gratitude has proven to be a significant cause of positive outcomes." Gratitude doesn't mean we won't get down or feel sad. No matter how blessed we are in our lives, we all experience sadness. These feelings don't mean we are ungrateful, and they are not a reason to shame ourselves. We berate ourselves with labels like "first-world problems" for what are often valid concerns. And yes, most of our problems are first-world, because that is where we live, and that is the perspective from which we see life and the place from which our problems arise. Therefore, it is important to validate our feelings and then come up with ways not to get caught in a ruminating spin cycle of negativity. One great way to do that is to focus on a couple of things we are grateful for in the moment. Gratitude is an anecdote to anxiety. Being grateful is a valuable tool to take care of our mind's health.

There is a helpful TED talk by researcher Guy Winch titled "Why We All Need to Practice Emotional First Aid." He observes that we spend a lot of time discussing our personal hygiene and physical health, while our mind—the cornerstone of our being—is left unattended and, worse yet, is abused by our negative self-talk. I have witnessed that tendency for myself in my work as a dietitian. The people I meet in my practice are, on the whole, smart, driven, interesting, and kind. Yet the story they tell themselves is that they are lazy, weak, and not good enough. Those messages work against us, not for us. Learning to love ourselves is a tall order, and appreciating our strengths is not akin to giving up on our aspirations. We are incredibly hard on ourselves, and we set standards that we would never expect of someone else. Think about the mean things we say in our heads to and about ourselves: "I am so stupid." "Why do I even bother?" "I am such an idiot." "I can't do anything right." "I'll never accomplish my goals." Now think about replacing each of those "I's" with "you." Worse yet, think about making those statements to your children. Never. We would never demoralize them like that. Why? Because we would harm their sense of self, and make them feel rejected and not good enough. And we know that's not the way to help people reach their potential. Saying it to ourselves is not any better. It is time to work on treating ourselves with the love and respect that we deserve. The results will be life changing.

We have now covered three foundational pieces in the Pyramid to Healthy Eating. Read these sections as many times as necessary to bolster your resolve to Ditch the Diet, and to work on the skills that form the cornerstone of the healthy and happy life you deserve. When you truly focus on mindfulness surrounding eating, relax some of the food rules we all get caught up in, begin to accept your body enough to live in your skin, then you can move into building new habits with nutritional shifts that fit your life.

Putting It into Practice

What are your personal challenges to accepting your body?

What mantras or personal affirmations will you choose that may help you overcome those challenges?

Chapter 10
Create Lasting Habits

Affirmation: I value progress, not perfection.

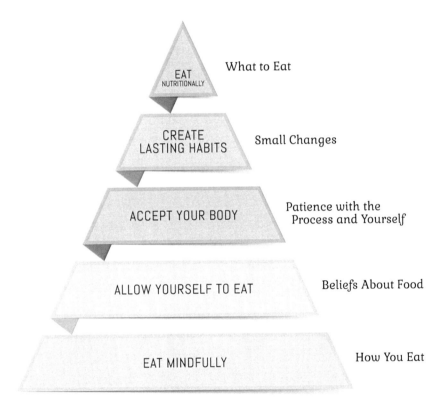

EAT
NUTRITIONALLY — What to Eat

CREATE
LASTING HABITS — Small Changes

ACCEPT YOUR BODY — Patience with the Process and Yourself

ALLOW YOURSELF TO EAT — Beliefs About Food

EAT MINDFULLY — How You Eat

WE HAVE REACHED the fourth level of the Pyramid to Healthy Eating, where we will focus on creating lasting habits. It's time to delve into the importance of making small changes and building wellness behaviors that lead to lifelong health. As we work our way through this chapter, let's keep the above affirmation at the forefront: we should value *progress*, not *perfection*. Recognizing that this is a process and celebrating the small wins will help provide the peace of mind to stay the course. What I have found with my clients is that there is an "aha moment" when this mind shift takes place, when they realize that they can make positive changes, still enjoy food, and feel good about themselves—all while living life. When the realization occurs, I can almost feel the huge weight being lifted from them.

As I continue to emphasize throughout this chapter, taking this journey one step at a time will yield the lifelong results you are working toward. We are establishing habits, and that requires time, patience, and a commitment to both moderation and consistency. This isn't a box you check and then move on; this is the long haul where you settle in and embrace the ebb and flow. You have Ditched the Diet, and the days of agonizing over what you can or can't eat are over.

The research on habits has made some exciting advances as we learn more about how our brain works, where habits form, and how to manipulate them. We do a lot of things without even thinking about it. Some of those things we consider good habits and others we wish we could extinguish. A primitive part of our brain called the basal ganglia is responsible for this, allowing us to do things even if we have no memory for how to do them. Once a habit is formed, it is widely accepted that it will lurk in our brain for good. However, if it is a habit we don't want, there are ways to replace it with something new. In his book *The Power of Habit*, Charles Duhigg explains habits as a loop consisting of a cue, the routine, and the reward. The research he presents is brilliantly laid out, and his writing weaves the research, stories, and application together in a way that is accessible and understandable. One of the take-home messages about changing habits is that if you identify the cue and the reward for the habit, you can replace the routine using that same cue and reward. Therefore, to go about making a change, first you want to determine the stimulus or cue that initiates a particular habit or routine. It can be almost anything: a visual trigger, a time of day, a place, a certain activity, an emotion, thoughts, certain people … you get the idea. That cue initiates the routine, and then the routine elicits a particular reward.

What is the reward you receive for a particular habit? It can be a physical sensation, or maybe it is an emotional payoff, such as a feeling of pride. Once you have identified the cue for the routine and the reward that you get from the routine, then you can change the routine. The next step is to come up with a different routine that you can do when exposed to the same cue, and it should have the same reward. The "Putting It into Practice" worksheet at the end of this chapter will help walk you through this process for yourself.

It is interesting to consider how our brain physically makes adjustments that allow us to follow through with responses to certain cues even without consciously thinking about it. The more often we do a certain routine, the more ingrained and automatic it becomes. This works both in the formation of negative habits, like automatically looking at a text when we hear the ding regardless of what we are doing, to helping us reach goals we are actively pursuing, like drinking water as soon as we wake up in the morning. Not only are we using positive cognitions to teach ourselves a new skill, but our brains are also rewarding our tenacity biologically. Since created habits are stored in the brain, it is always possible for old habits to finagle their way back in. However, by being conscious of that possibility, you can identify when it happens and actively work to replace it again.

Obstacles and challenges might arise in habit building, tempting us to drop a new skill or activity. But persevering and problem-solving through this period are important. Our new habit will become a combined result of learning and building! I have noticed in my own life that as I move past a couple weeks of a new routine, new obstacles arise that I have to work around. It takes determination to keep on keeping on. Sure, there are always valid excuses not to continue a positive activity, but staying resolute will give us more flexibility in the future. Once those pathways have been formed in the brain, we have an added boost to pick back up a good habit even when we've skipped it here and there. The longer we stick to something, the greater the chance of retention, an idea that reinforces this book's underlying premises of being patient, taking it slow, and doing things consistently.

All this research about creating habits makes it sound so straightforward and almost easy; yet the nitty-gritty of forming new habits is hard. We sometimes complicate matters by fooling ourselves into believing that we are sticking to a good habit more consistently than we really are. We say, "I've been exercising every day for the past three months," because that was the goal and we like to believe we are meeting that goal. However, if we tracked our daily activity, we might notice we are averaging more like four days per week. So, as you challenge yourself to build new habits, you must be realistic and honest to set yourself up for success. Let's look at some tips and ideas for effective habit building when it comes to nutrition.

Choose a Healthy and Achievable Habit

The big question becomes: what nutritionally healthy habits do we want to establish? To create a lasting habit, it needs to be a good one to begin with, and something that doesn't work against our body, mind, and human nature. We will be looking at specific nutrition recommendations when we arrive at the tip of the Pyramid to Healthy Eating in the next chapter, which is all about eating nutritionally. For now, let's focus on building healthy habits.

It is important to recognize that even when you create habits in a healthy and manageable way, they are still a lifelong commitment. And yet habits, even when established, will still ebb and flow over time. Our lives are too multifaceted for routines to be completely rigid and static. Even though a habit may have been established for a commendable period of time, we may occasionally need to give ourselves a reality check and reboot a habit that has fallen off. Often, while giving presentations, I preface a piece of nutritional information with, "Now you probably already know this, but let's talk about it again." That's because most great information bears repeating, not to mention hearing it from various perspectives and at different times. We can only take in so much information at a time, and we gravitate toward the pieces that we can assimilate at any moment. We may have heard all the advice, yet one idea spoke to us today. Then a year later we review our notes and find a totally different nugget of helpful information.

Even for me, a professional dietitian, I need to find ways to stay engaged with good nutrition information and apply it to a regular routine. That's something we all need to do, no matter where we are in our nutritional journey. Not only do we want to establish habits that are moderate, truly healthy, and doable, but we also need to make a habit of regularly reviewing good, new information. That may look different for each of us. You could follow a helpful nutrition blog or Facebook page, or read research journals. Maybe you enjoy flipping through cookbooks or receiving newsletters with healthy insights. Consider listening to podcasts while driving, doing chores, or exercising. Whatever you choose, you will find that plugging into reputable nutrition resources is motivating and helpful in your daily quest for wellness.

Track Your Habits to Help Change Them

Habit tracking is an objective and concrete tool that, when used consistently and appropriately, can help to effect valuable change. Writing down a habit serves as both a motivator and a form of accountability—both highly important qualities when trying to create new habits. Tracking also gives you a record of what you have accomplished, regardless of the final outcome. What is the best way to track a habit? As with anything, the answer will partially depend on your personality, but I'm going to lay out a few ideas and tenets to keep in mind, no matter which method you decide to try.

Set an action-oriented goal, and write it down in a place where you can look at it a few times each day. Then create the action items that will allow you to attain that goal; your action items also become activities you will track. This will look something like this:

Action-oriented goal:
I will eat three servings of vegetables per day.

Action items:
1. Cut up an assortment of vegetables on Sunday.
2. Eat at least one serving at breakfast or lunch.
3. Find a new way to prepare a vegetable and plan a time to try it.

Find a platform, such as a spreadsheet or notebook, for recording your action items as you complete them. This book has an appendix labeled "Ditch the Diet Habit Tracker," where you will find a habit-tracking spreadsheet that you can copy, download from my website, and fill out on your computer or print and write on. I include a couple of size options, so that if you decide to print a copy, you can choose what works best with your system. For instance, the 8-x-10 size could slip into a binder, folder, or pad folio that you use daily, or hang on a bulletin board or refrigerator in your home or office. Meanwhile, the smaller size could slide or tape into a planner or journal, or become a bookmark for a book you are reading.

Be intentional about filling in your habit-tracking chart. Tracking is yet another habit to be instituted (yes, we have to create a new habit in order to stick to our other new habits!). Actually, it shouldn't be difficult if you are purposeful about marking an action when you do it. That may also alert you to other listed activities you still need to accomplish that day or week.

Although I've been using a tracking chart for a while now, I still find its power to be shocking. Realizing that I still have a box or two to mark has a weird influence over me. Sure, I might be annoyed about complying with my task, and I have been known to complain and grumble; but most of the time, when I am tracking something, I feel I had better follow through. Sometimes, I look at my chart and say, "Forget about it; not going to happen today." When you have those same thoughts, I want you to know it is okay! Perfection is not our goal, remember? But for the most part, the chart can be a helpful tool for accountability.

Stack Your Habits

Pair a new habit with an old one. There is evidence to suggest that one way to help create a new habit is to "stack it" with something you already do readily in your life, such as brushing your teeth, using the restroom, or hitting send on an e-mail. For example, if your goal is to drink 64 ounces of water per day, then one of your action steps could be to have a sip of water every time you send an e-mail. Part of the difficulty with creating new habits is figuring out the logistics of when and how, as well as remembering to do it. If you are stacking it with an existing behavior or routine, then you have some of the difficulty resolved. Basically we are using the cue for an established habit, behavior, or activity to double as the cue for a new habit. What a clever way to get more bang for your buck!

Pace Yourself

Don't embark on too many goals at once. Remember that we are trying to help our brain create a healthy habit that will eventually become ingrained in our life without having to constantly think about it. That may be more difficult to achieve if we are tackling too much. I know that it seems tedious to have to pull back when we are so motivated to fix our whole life all at once. Yet we know that it doesn't work out in the long run to do it that way. We have learned this lesson repeatedly—at least once a year with the dawn of the New Year and all the life-perfecting goals that we so sincerely set for ourselves. I get it, and I feel the tug, too! It seems so easy in theory, and a string of 5 to 10 goals covering all areas of our lives seems really doable—especially this year, we tell ourselves, because somehow it is going to work out better this time. Does this self-talk sound similar to what we say to ourselves when we begin a new diet? Here is an example of some New Year's goals that I would love to institute:

Nutrition: Eat five servings of vegetables every day.
Exercise: Do 10 minutes of yoga before bed every night.
Spirituality: Read a family devotion each evening at dinner.
Financial: Log every daily expense before bedtime.
Career: Read and tweet one relevant research article each morning.
Personal: Volunteer once a month with a social justice organization.

I tell myself that I should already be practicing these goals and that it really isn't that much to institute. My list seems as if it should be doable—but in fact it is too much, especially considering all the things in each category that I already do on a regular basis. If we want to achieve long-term goals and build lifelong habits, we need to keep it manageable and realistic.

In the next chapter you will read all about nutrition and the many ways we can eat to enhance our health. This is where it can be tempting to tackle *all* the things. I encourage you to institute new goals in your life one at a time, making each one relevant to your current life, and committing to consistency and problem solving along the way. Then move on to another one. It is always good to maintain a list of goals and aspirations, because keeping those ideas in our consciousness will help make them a reality someday, as long as we tackle them one by one. If you focus on a single goal at a time and really sink your teeth into each one, then you're more likely to figure out how to make it a lifelong habit.

Reexamine a New Habit

The tactics we employ to maintain a new habit may need to be different at different phases in our lives. This is why it is important to make a practice of periodically reviewing how our healthy behaviors are working for us. Go back and review some of your goals and aspirations for maintaining a healthy lifestyle, and reexamine how your current routines are matching up. One way to do this with respect to nutrition standards is to keep a food journal for one to three days. For example, if one of your healthy habits is to have a piece of fruit with breakfast every day, a journal will let you see how well that is panning out. More information about food journaling is coming up in chapter 12.

It is important to keep in mind the transience of life when you realize that things just are not working like they used to. Take a look at what is going on in your life right now, and compare it to how your life looked when things seemed smoother. Maybe you have a new commitment or schedule that makes your old ways less feasible now, which is why a certain discipline keeps falling through the cracks. I have become very aware of how frequently the patterns of my life change depending on the different stages that my children and family are in. The advantage is that each season brings new possibilities. Choices that were not available a year ago are all of a sudden a miraculous option today. Being open-minded and willing to try new ways of tackling a problem can lead to pleasant surprises.

MY NEW HABIT

This chapter has covered five tips that should help give you the tools to build lasting habits over time: choose a habit that is healthy and achievable; track it; stack it; pace yourself; and then reexamine it once it's been in place for a while. Now let me turn the focus on me for a moment, and how I had to establish a new habit in order to write this book. As I share my story, notice how I employed my own tips in creating this new routine in my life.

Writing this book has been an interesting experiment in many different ways. The insights, lessons, and take-home messages I've gained have been unexpected. As you will see, until I made a conscious effort to form a new habit to facilitate my writing process, the progress of my book was much slower and emotionally draining. Getting the jumble of ideas, concepts, and information from my brain into coherent words on paper has been dramatically more difficult than I ever imagined. The process required a diversity of skill sets that surely don't come naturally to any one person. It has been a completely paradoxical experience involving both creativity and gut-wrenching self-discipline, flexibility and rigidity, attention to detail and the ability to think abstractly, seeing things from multiple perspectives yet narrowing the scope to a meaningful answer. The problem solving that I've had to do has come with a lot of trial and error, and ironically has added content to this book, as I discovered things to help myself that will also help my clients and to you.

However, as we all know, when something is difficult, it can be tempting to procrastinate. After a few years of trying to write this book, I realized one of my primary problems: I continually let other obligations take precedence over my writing. In order to change that habit, I had to institute a totally different routine. Instead of going into my office in the morning and checking e-mail and phone messages and getting caught up in the to-do lists of the day, I began going straight to the local Starbucks at 8 a.m. after dropping children at school. In the hour and a half I stayed there, I didn't log onto the Internet, check e-mail, or look at my phone. I only wrote. If words didn't come, I stared into space and listened to the murmurings of strangers until I had some meaningful thoughts. Some days produced more writing results than others, but each day contributed to a beneficial routine that has ultimately made all the difference. Now, that hour and a half of writing is marked on my calendar, and I consider it as firm an obligation as I would a scheduled client.

There are so many valuable resources out there on building habits that would make wonderful additions to the five tips I covered here. Those resources may also provide additional insight into the psychology of habit forming, procrastination, and the mental games that we play with ourselves. The message I hope you take away from this chapter is that you can do this. Make measurable, moderate changes and recognize that change takes time. And don't beat yourself up in the process. As you climb the Pyramid to Healthy Eating, knowing how to build healthy habits in a moderate and achievable manner will allow you to choose nutritional goals that are right for you, and will help you implement them in your life.

Putting It into Practice

In this exercise, let's think through Charles Duhigg's explanation of habits, shown below:

Cue → Routine → Reward

Write down a routine or a habit that you have. (My example: I drink a glass of water from my nightstand as soon as I wake up in the morning.)

What is the cue that initiates that routine or habit? (My example: My alarm goes off to wake me up.)

What reward do you get from completing that routine/habit? (My example: My mouth feels better, it helps to wake me up a little bit, and I feel good about doing something healthy for my body.)

Now use that same cue-routine-reward system to establish a new routine or replace a less desirable habit with a new one. Think about both the cue for the habit and the reward that you get from it:

Cue:

Reward:

Now consider inserting a new routine that will give you the same reward:
Routine:

Chapter 11
Eat Nutritionally

Affirmation: I enjoy lots of different foods.

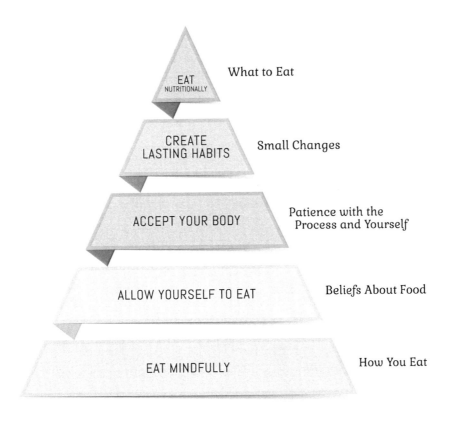

EAT NUTRITIONALLY — What to Eat

CREATE LASTING HABITS — Small Changes

ACCEPT YOUR BODY — Patience with the Process and Yourself

ALLOW YOURSELF TO EAT — Beliefs About Food

EAT MINDFULLY — How You Eat

THIS IS THE MOMENT you have been waiting for! We have now reached the top of the Pyramid to Healthy Eating and the pinnacle of our process: eating nutritionally. We are finally going to talk about what to eat and why. Most diets are made up entirely of what to eat, but for us this is the cherry on top. You have by now established a solid foundation for how to eat, which moved you through the stages encouraging you to: eat mindfully, allow yourself to eat, accept your body, and create lasting habits. You are now ready to focus on what to eat. And we can do so with the confidence that it will enhance our health all the way around.

Here we will focus on foods and nutrition that have strong, evidence-based benefits, and strategies for incorporating them into the diet. Nutrition choices look different for everyone.

Intake of certain foods may decrease for some people, while increasing for others. We will constantly strive to increase the variety in our diet by trying new foods and recipes, and coming up with unique ideas for healthy meals that can vary each day. We will use techniques that increase acceptance and love of ourselves as we improve our health, energy, and happiness by making slow, measured habit changes.

In my private practice, I frequently offer opportunities for my clients and my followers to participate in wellness challenges at certain integral times of the year. This is one of the most popular things I do one-on-one with clients and also indirectly through social media. In these challenges, I prepare lists of activities for participants to accomplish each day, activities intended to be a manageable way to create new habits. I get them to focus on a couple of key nutrition concepts so that they are not trying to change everything at the same time. These challenges have posed an interesting challenge for me as well, since it requires me to give general advice that will be helpful to groups of people while also stressing the importance of always tailoring goals to each individual. It's a pretty tall order, and I have found that, when it comes to changes and challenges, smaller is better.

This chapter addresses a whole host of nutritional goals you can aspire to. I have provided sample goals at the end of each section to give you some direction. Yet I want to encourage you to develop your own goals as you go along and to incorporate them into your life gradually. As with all the steps we have covered in this book, you should never try to take on too much all at once.

Water

Sometimes the simplest things have the greatest impact, which is why I am opening our discussion of nutritional choices with a basic need: water. I'm not sure why, but I can get resistance from clients when I tell them the importance of drinking enough water each day. Maybe the perception is that the payoff can't be all that great, or maybe chronic dieters believe that they should tackle a bigger and better nutritional goal. However, staying properly hydrated has a wide range of benefits, which I list below. Water has become the first place I turn if I am not feeling quite right, and it's also the answer I give my kids when they come to me with an ailment. By now, they're so accustomed to my water prescription that they preface any complaint with "Mom, I already drank some water, but …" Because our bodies use water to accomplish almost every function, hydration is a crucial part of staying healthy. Here are just a few reasons why drinking enough water is important:

- o   Our body is mostly water.
- o   Water heals.
- o   Water regulates body temperature (and, as it gets hotter, you need more).
- o   Water keeps mucous membranes moist and fluid; thin mucous helps with upper respiratory congestion.

o   Water flushes our system of toxins, and keeps bowels moving and healthy.

o   Water cushions our joints, which helps prevent injury and pain.

o   Mild dehydration is a common cause of headaches and migraines, and proper water intake may decrease the duration of headaches and incidences of onset.

o   Proper hydration will improve energy levels (80 percent of our population may suffer energy loss due to minor dehydration).

o   Water will decrease muscle aches.

o   Proper hydration helps in the management of depression and chronic fatigue syndrome.

o   Often thirst can be confused with hunger. We might choose a snack when what we really need is water.

To help determine how much water an individual should drink each day, I have a ballpark formula I like to use. The simple formula is to take your body weight in pounds and divide by two. This number will give you the number of ounces of water to drink per day. For example, if you take a person who weighs 150 pounds and divide that by two, then that equals 75 ounces of water per day. Again, this is a general formula that needs to be adjusted based on individual differences and requirements. One indicator to determine if your water intake is on target is the color of your urine. Pale yellow (like lemonade) is the goal. If your urine is clear, drink less water; and if it is dark yellow, drink more. I recommend you listen to your body and adjust your water intake accordingly. If you find that too much water at once makes you feel nauseous or sloshes around in your stomach, then back off. (It is usually better to drink water consistently versus chugging 32 ounces twice a day.) Play with patterns that work for you. Hydration may need to be adjusted according to the seasons, heat, humidity/aridity, the fluid content of food intake, and so on. And sometimes your body requires more electrolytes in addition to water to account for sweat losses. Here are some tips for staying on target with water consumption:

o   Carry a refillable water bottle with you everywhere, in a size that works for you.

o   Choose water with meals.

o   Drink water during workouts.

o   For a head start on the day and to replace overnight water losses, keep 8–12 ounces of water next to your bed and drink it upon waking up in the morning.

o   Set a timer to go off periodically as a reminder to take a sip of water and stretch.

o   Take regular medications with 10–20 ounces of water.

o   Cut fresh lemons/cucumber/mint and add to your water bottle.

By increasing water in your diet, you may find that it displaces other choices that are not as healthy or nourishing for your body, such as soda or energy drinks. As you become more steadily hydrated, your taste for water will increase. You will crave it! You may worry that increasing your water intake will make you have to use the bathroom too often. Another interesting anecdote is that after a few weeks of increased water intake, your bladder will adjust so that you will go less often but with more volume.

Goal
Do you need to drink more water? If so, choose this as one of your goals. Here's an idea:
> *Choose two or three of the hydration tips from the previous list, and then create some specific action items to achieve them.*

Fruits and Vegetables

The importance of fruits and vegetables in your daily diet cannot be overstated. If you want to improve wellness, this is where to start—and I can almost say this unilaterally, for every eater in every situation. Fruits and vegetables are high in fiber, phytochemicals, vitamins, and minerals, all of which have a wide scope of benefits which we will discuss in detail in this section. The goal for a healthy diet is to eat five to nine servings of fruits and vegetables each day. Many days I absolutely do not make it to that goal. It takes a conscious effort for all of us, myself included, to get enough fruits and vegetables in our diets, especially in this age of hurried lives, busy schedules, and convenience foods. Even though it's hard to maintain consistency, we still need to make fruits and vegetables a nutritional habit that we stay aware of. The ebb and flow of life will create an ebb and flow in your food intake, and you can't eat perfectly every day. That's okay, though you should keep good nutritional choices present in your mind as much as possible. If you have a few crazy days without a single vegetable at all, then your mind ought to tell you to fit in some veggies the next time you have a little leeway in your schedule.

The value of vegetables is indisputable, even in most fad diets. When we look at fad diets, there are generally two common denominators: they tend to be restricted in calories and bountiful in vegetables. I don't think that any fad diet would dare to vilify vegetables. That might well be the kiss of death for the diet provocateur's pocketbook. Yet I take offense at some of the ways the vegetables are recommended in many fad diets, with only certain vegetables "allowed" or having to be prepared a specific way. Vegetables are beneficial, period, whether they are cooked, raw, frozen, canned, and whether you eat them with salt, butter, dressing, or plain. The value of the vegetable remains. And different preparation techniques will add to the variety of your meals and the resulting benefits. Now, of course I am not suggesting canned green beans drenched in butter with every meal for a person with heart disease. And someone with diabetes will need to pay attention to their portion size of certain vegetables. Additionally, a person suffering with IBS may avoid certain vegetables to manage symptoms. All these scenarios are individualized, and even within a group of people with the same disease to manage, each person's food plan will look different. You have to figure out what your own dietary needs are, and use common sense when making your nutritional goals. Yet, a fad diet recommendation for everyone to eat only raw vegetables, for example, is not good advice to extrapolate to the whole population.

Fruit is also an essential and integral component of a well-rounded healthy diet, yet is sometimes vilified by the fad diet contingent. Why? Because of its natural sugar. As the bad rap surrounding sugar intensifies, then the quick solution for our extremist society is to cut out fruits completely. But that's a bad idea, because fruit is much more than its sugar content (and, by the way, sugar is an integral component of metabolism). Fruit also contributes fiber, phytochemicals, vitamins, and minerals—just like the vegetables. And because of its natural sugar content, fruit is a wonderful and healthy form of energy. Plus, fruit tastes good. Because many people prefer it, I often advise picky eaters that don't like vegetables (and that means both children and their parents) to double up on their servings of fruits, as both food groups provide similar health benefits.

FIBER

Fiber is one of the components of fruits and vegetables that contributes to their health benefits. The average American gets about 11 grams of fiber per day. That's less than half of the recommended 25 to 35 grams. We have work to do when it comes to fiber. Adequate fiber in the diet has been found to have a whole host of health benefits. Not only does fiber help maintain bowel health and normalize bowel movements, but it also lowers cholesterol levels and rates of coronary heart disease, helps control blood sugar levels, and increases insulin sensitivity. A high fiber diet also increases immune support and mineral absorption (especially calcium), as well as decreasing hemorrhoid risk. It is also possible that a high fiber diet decreases the risk of colorectal cancer.

Fiber is found in two forms, soluble and insoluble, each contributing to the health benefits listed above. Some of the best sources of fiber are fruits, vegetables, whole grains, and legumes/beans. And if you get a wide variety of those foods, then you will cover the bases of both sources of fiber. Sure, fiber can be found as an additive in bars, smoothies, and supplements, but the gold standard is to get it from whole foods. Once we start ratcheting up that fiber figure with supplements like inulin and chicory root, we may be opening a new can of worms. Learn more about additional sources of high fiber foods in the upcoming section on "Whole Grains and Fiber."

But do not attempt to increase your fiber all at once, or you will not feel good. Start with an additional five grams per day for one to two weeks, being sure to also drink plenty of water. Then, once your body has adjusted to that amount, you can up your fiber level again in the same manner. This should temper any undue stomach discomfort, unless you suffer with other gastrointestinal ailments such as IBS. In that case, it is important to seek counsel from an RDN specializing in this field in order to facilitate the process of finding tolerable fiber foods (see Appendix A on where to find good nutrition information).

PHYTOCHEMICALS

Phytochemicals are elements that are present in all fruits and vegetables and beans and grains. There have been more than 4,000 identified with about 150 studied in depth. In short, phytochemicals are the chemicals that make up the defense shield for a plant. Every plant has different phytochemicals, and when we consume various plant foods (fruits, vegetables, grains, nuts, seeds, legumes, herbs), we get benefits from their phytochemicals as well. Some of the ways they benefit us include decreasing risk of certain cancers, protecting against heart disease, providing anti-inflammatory properties, and strengthening the immune system. As research continues and methods for assessing phytochemical benefits improve, we continue to learn even more. One discovery is that there is a synergistic effect when getting the phytochemical from its natural food source versus in a supplement form. This may be due to the interactions between the naturally occurring fiber, vitamins, and other nutrients in the food with the phytochemical component. Another interesting side note is how certain phytochemicals are more bioavailable once cooked or processed. For example, the benefit of the phytochemical lycopene, found in tomato products, is more potent from processed tomatoes such as canned tomatoes, salsa, ketchup, and tomato sauce, than from a raw whole tomato. However, the raw tomato is still an important health asset because in that form it will provide more of such nutrients as vitamin A and C than will its processed counterpart.

While it can be difficult to isolate a specific phytochemical and its corresponding benefit, the research is ongoing and there is strong evidence for some correlations. For example, lycopene, which is found in tomatoes as well as other orange, yellow, and red plants, may be associated with a decreased risk of prostate cancer. And anthocyanins, a subclass of the flavonoid group, found in cherries, blueberries, and acai to name a few, helps decrease inflammation in the body and protect against atherosclerosis. Other classes of flavonoids found in fruits, tea, wine, cocoa, and soybeans also contribute to these same protections, as well as having anti-diabetic activities. Resveratrol found in red wine, grapes, peanuts, and some berries may provide cardiovascular protection and boast anti-inflammatory and anticancer properties.

The above examples barely scratch the surface when discussing all the potential benefits and the ongoing research being done with phytochemicals. The diversity of metabolic mechanisms at play is quite astounding. Your best course of action is to eat a variety of plant foods prepared in a variety of ways. Mix it up, eat your fruits and veggies in various forms, and try lots of different ones in order to incorporate many different phytochemicals in your diet.

VITAMINS AND MINERALS

Another component of fruits and vegetables that make them so valuable is their vitamin and mineral content. They are packed with essential vitamins and minerals. Essential means that our body cannot make them, and therefore we have to get vitamins and minerals from the foods they are in. We could take a ton of vitamins in supplement form—and many of us do, almost like purchasing a good insurance policy on our health. However, supplements will never provide as complete a benefit as eating the foods that contain those vitamins and minerals. Sure, it is helpful that we have access to vitamins and minerals in supplement form. There are situations when that resource is a life saver. However, when the whole food is available, the value of eating it is more far-reaching than a supplement form. Some vitamins and minerals work well together and enhance each other's absorption, while some impede it. When eating a variety of whole foods, these interactions tend to even out. By contrast, when you rely on supplements, those nuances can make eating into a complicated science.

The take-home message for vegetables and fruits is that they are very healthy, packed with nutrients, and strong disease fighters. They should make up a substantial portion of our overall diet. Again, we are individuals with varying needs, genetics, and histories, so some of our specific food choices will vary. We should choose from a variety of fruits and veggies, and eat them daily. Pick the ones you most enjoy and tolerate. Prepare them in ways that are palatable to you, and also meet the standards for your personal health picture.

Goal

Do you need to increase your fruit and vegetable intake? Here are a couple of ways you might try to do this:

> *Eat four to five servings of vegetables per day, making sure that one serving comes from a green leafy source.*
> *Have one serving of fruit with breakfast each day.*

Whole Grains and Fiber

When we consider that the average person needs 50 percent of his or her total calorie intake to come from carbohydrates, then the value of grains cannot be overstated. As covered in an earlier chapter, carbohydrates are important for a multitude of reasons—energy for our brain, body, and muscles being just one. And one very valuable source of carbohydrates in the diet is grains, such as rice, quinoa, wheat, barley, bread, cereal, pasta, and oats. Not only do these grains provide us with energy, but they are also great plant-based sources of fiber, phytochemicals, vitamins, and minerals, among other things. Is this beginning to sound familiar? Yes, because we also get some of these same benefits from fruits and vegetables. So why not just eat fruits and veggies? Why do we need these grains anyway? Well, for one, they taste great. They add unique textures and chewiness to meals, which is an important contribution to helping make food satisfying. They also have specific phytochemicals, vitamins, and minerals that no other foods can provide. They are not quite as bulky as fruits and vegetables, so they can provide healthy calories in smaller portions. If we were eating just vegetables and fruits, then to get enough calories we would have to eat them all day long.

What does an appropriate grain intake for optimal health look like? It can be slightly different for everyone, but this illustration provides a good starting place:

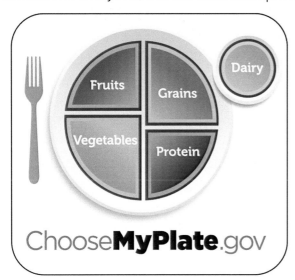

You see that one quarter of this plate is dedicated to grains, and ideally we would like those grains to include *whole* grains. So, where do whole grains fit in, and what exactly are they? Whole grains are the grain products that still contain most of their original fiber and nutrient content. In other words, the original product has not been processed and refined to a point at which it has lost most of its original fiber. A few examples of whole grains include:

- Whole wheat bread, pasta, or crackers
- Whole grain cereals
- Brown and wild rice
- Popcorn
- Old-fashioned oats
- Quinoa
- Bulgur
- Barley
- Rye

Of our total grain intake, a good objective is to get half from whole grain sources. Make it feasible and enjoyable based on your individual circumstances, likes, and dislikes. For example, maybe you enjoy whole wheat bread for your sandwiches and toast, and you like brown rice as much as white in a stir-fry, but you draw the line at whole wheat pasta. Fine. Make that work. Take a look at your snack foods, too, and remember that choices do not have to be static. Most of the time you may be satisfied with the wheat crackers, but sometimes the only thing that will do are classic potato chips! Remember that life fluctuates, and so do our food choices. It is going to be fine.

Goal

Do you want to focus on whole grains and fiber? Try this:

> *Track the fiber content in your meals for two to three days. If you are below the*
> *recommended 25 grams per day, see if there are some places where you can substitute*
> *a higher fiber alternative, trying to add about 5 grams of fiber to your daily total.*

Omega 3s and Fats

Fat is amazing—and it's one of my all-time favorite topics. First of all, it makes things taste great. Second, it has stellar health benefits. Note that this section is titled "Omega 3s and Fats," because many Americans are lacking the omega 3 fatty acids in their diets. These have so many health benefits and fit significantly into a larger picture of dietary fats.

Let's start with a lesson on fat and clear up some misconceptions. Most importantly, fat in food does not translate to fat on the body—unless you have more calories than you need for the day. If that's the case, it doesn't matter where the calories come from; the excess can come from fat, protein, or carbohydrates, but it will be stored as fat in the body. So, if all you eat is protein, but the total amount of protein consumed has more calories than your body can process, it would be stored as fat. The only way that reducing fat in the diet will reduce fat on the body is if you don't make up those calories somewhere else. And since fat helps us feel satisfied, reducing it in the diet too much can leave us with hunger pangs and cravings.

As we discussed in chapter 8, "Allow Yourself to Eat," the recommended percentage of fat needed for an overall healthy diet is 20 to 35 percent of total calories. Now let's discuss the different types of fat, where these fats are found in food, and how they relate to our overall health. Keep in mind: labeling the fat within a food as saturated or unsaturated, or as polyunsaturated or monounsaturated (we will discuss all these terms below), is a generalization about the majority component of the fat in that food. Most food sources of fat in our diets include all the types of fat, just in varying ratios. I've included a chart, Comparison of Dietary Fats, to illustrate this point.

Saturated fat, for the most part, includes the fats that are solid at room temperature. Think butter, lard, and the marbling in meat. Current recommendations are that less than 10 percent of our total calorie intake should come from saturated fat. That's because levels higher than that are related to high LDL (bad) cholesterol levels and an increased risk of heart disease.

Unsaturated fat, on the other hand, is the fat that is liquid at room temperature. This can be in the form of plant-based oils such as olive oil, safflower oil, or grapeseed oil or within foods like avocados, nuts, and olives, to name a few. If saturated fat makes up 10 percent of our daily calorie intake, then that leaves 10 to 25 percent to come from unsaturated sources. These fats have many health benefits attributed to them, as we will see.

Unsaturated fat can be broken down further into polyunsaturated fatty acids (PUFA) and monounsaturated fatty acids (MUFA). Both of these fats are considered to be cardio protective when in the proper amounts and ratios. The diet of people in the Mediterranean region has

Comparison of Dietary Fats

Dietary Fat

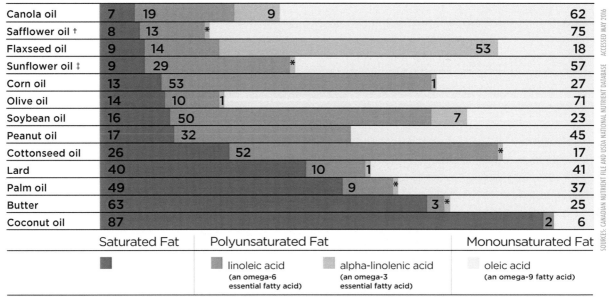

† High Oleic ‡ Mid Oleic * Trace   Fatty acid content expressed as g/100g fat

With permission from the Canola Council of Canada

been extensively researched, and it has been noted that the high consumption of MUFAs in that culture correlates to a very low incidence of heart disease. Many other components of the Mediterranean diet have added health benefits as well, such as the whole grain base, voluminous amounts of fruits and vegetables, and meat as an accent versus a centerpiece, all combined with an active lifestyle.

Some foods that are high in MUFAs include:

o   Olives and olive oil
o   Avocados
o   Nuts and nut butters
o   Safflower oil
o   Canola oil
o   Sesame oil

Polyunsaturated fats (PUFAs) are also valuable to our health; however, we have discovered a caveat here. PUFA can be broken down into further categories, two of which are omega 6 fatty acids and omega 3 fatty acids. The caveat is that the greatest benefit comes when these two fats are in a favorable ratio, even as close as 1:1. Various diseases see benefits at 2:1 to 5:1 of omega 6 to omega 3. Yet most of us are far off of that mark. In fact, the ratio in Western diets is currently estimated at 15:1 to 17:1. Omega 6 fatty acids are an essential fat needed by the body, yet they are usually consumed in large quantities in the typical American diet; so, to regulate the ratio, we are encouraged to increase omega 3 fats in the diet. The greatest benefits from improving this ratio appear to surround cardiovascular disease, cancer, inflammatory processes, and immune diseases. Some foods that are high in omega 3 fatty acids include:

- o Fatty fish such as salmon, tuna, mackerel, herring, whitefish, trout, sardines
- o Walnuts
- o Flaxseed
- o Pumpkin seeds
- o Wheat germ

It is fair to say that almost everyone can benefit from increasing the amount of omega 3 fatty acids in their diet. This is a first line of defense in my practice for those suffering from inflammation, which is connected to practically all health issues.

Goal

Do you want to work on increasing healthy fats in your diet? Try this:

Eat one serving of fish two times a week, and choose one item from either of the above lists to have on the other days of the week.

Breakfast

Chapter 3 explains the importance of breakfast as it relates to our metabolism. If you need a refresher, go back and review those pages. In this section we will go into a little more detail about some additional benefits of breakfast and ways to incorporate it into your life on a consistent basis. Breakfast is vital for optimal wellness, so you should make it a priority to make it happen. It is a simple task that packs a lot of power.

First, as the name "breakfast" implies, this meal in the morning is breaking the fast that our body has been on while we slept. It is singlehandedly kick-starting a large piece of our metabolism (the Resting Metabolic Rate, or RMR) as well as contributing to the Thermic Effect of Feeding component of our metabolism that we covered in chapter 3. When you eat breakfast, you give your metabolism something to work on first thing in the morning. If you have a high-fiber, minimally processed, well-rounded breakfast, then your metabolism must work even harder.

Starting with a solid breakfast will also initiate the trend for eating three meals per day with a snack or two as needed—and that is a healthy pattern for most adults. When you skip breakfast, you end up cramming all your calories into one or two meals. That means that while your body is hungry and not getting any calories, you are burning muscle for energy. And then you will be so hungry from skipping a meal that the calories you get the rest of the day exceed what you need, and are stored as fat.

In terms of nutrition standards, breakfast can be a powerful element. The typical American breakfast offers a lot of healthy, well-balanced choices. Consider some of the common choices in the list below, and notice how they incorporate many of the nutritional components we have discussed. (Appendix E has a recipe blueprint for some of these options.)

⅔–1 cup granola
¼ cup walnuts
1 cup milk (any variety)
Berries, peaches, or other fresh or dried fruit for nutrients and fiber

½–1 cup oatmeal made with any kind of milk (regular, almond, soy)
Nuts, chia seeds, fruit, honey, peanut butter for flavor and protein
(Try making overnight oats for a variation on the traditional hot oatmeal.)

½ cup Greek yogurt
¼ cup sliced almonds and granola
Chia seeds and/or ground flaxseeds
Honey or maple Syrup
Dried fruit

Omelet with:
1–2 eggs
Cheese
Green onions, mushrooms, peppers, spinach, or other veggies
Touch of ham, bacon, sausage, or tofu
Side of fresh berries

Power breakfast sandwich:
2 slices whole-wheat toast or English muffin with:
1 egg, 1 ounce ham, and 1 slice cheese
(Cook your egg with some spinach to add a veggie to your day.)
Side of 4-ounce juice or fresh fruit

Peanut butter–banana sandwich:
2 slices whole-wheat toast or English muffin with:
2 tablespoons peanut butter and banana slices
1 cup milk

Grits or home-fried potatoes topped with or with a side of:
1–2 eggs
Choice of cheese
Bacon, ham, or tofu
Spinach, peppers, zucchini, broccoli, olives, or chives
Side of fruit

Don't forget about smoothies, especially if you don't have a great appetite in the morning. Sometimes drinking our calories is more tolerable for fussy stomachs. (Appendix E also includes a blueprint for a fun variation on a smoothie.)

Breakfast is a perfect time to get a dose of fiber, fruit, protein, carbohydrates, and healthy fats. And it gives us a chance to add variety to our diet, which should always be a nutritional goal. If you don't already start your day with breakfast, I encourage you to make every effort to add it. Think about your morning routine and where breakfast might fit. Replace a superfluous morning habit with breakfast. For example, instead of scrolling through social media for 15 minutes, prepare and eat a quick meal. Consider when, how, and what you might choose to eat. You can even eat in two phases: have a quick bite at home, and then carry something portable with you for the car or office. Keep it up, and soon you won't be able to go without this first meal of the day.

Goal
Do you want to improve your consistency in eating breakfast? Here's an idea:

> *Buy the ingredients to make at least three different breakfasts over a two-week period, and come up with a plan for how you will prepare and eat one of them each day. See which ones you like best, and keep those in your regular breakfast rotation.*

Regular Meals

Now that you see the value of eating breakfast, let's look at regular meals. For the same reasons we shouldn't skip our morning meal, we do not want to skip the rest of the day's meals either. Of course, it may not be realistic to have every meal every day. We all know that life is crazy. But if one of your patterns involves skipping meals multiple times a week, then you need to put this on your list of goals to address at some point.

Skipping meals sets in motion a whole string of potential wellness blasters. Hunger is a primal mechanism, and it will not be easily deterred. Here are some of the detrimental ways hunger may win over wellness:

- o When we are hungry, we crave foods that are calorie dense because our body knows they will do the job efficiently and quickly. Calorie-dense foods are high in fat and sugar. So, when you skip lunch, the steamed vegetable and rice dinner suddenly loses its appeal, and ordering pizza becomes the new plan.

o   When you have skipped a meal and are hungry, you have a much greater tendency to eat fast. When you eat fast, you can stuff a lot more calories into your stomach before your brain has a chance to realize you were full 15 bites ago.

o   The nutrients we need—both macronutrients and micronutrients—aren't utilized as effectively when we get them all at once, as opposed to consuming them over three to four meals.

Goal

Are you skipping meals regularly? Make a new plan:

Begin with the meal that gets skipped most often, and consider the reason. Devise different solutions. The interfering factors can be so different from one person to another that the solutions need differ as well. Sometimes we don't take the time to eat because we are busy meeting other people's needs before our own. If that sounds familiar, consider taking small steps to put your own needs higher on the list.

All the Macronutrients

We discussed macronutrients in Chapter 8, "Allow Yourself to Eat," and here it is again! As a reminder, macronutrients are the three nutrients consumed in large quantities that provide the energy we need: carbohydrates, protein, and fat. We need to eat all three macronutrients every single day. As a nutritionist, sometimes I take this knowledge for granted, and many RDNs may do the same; it is one of the core concepts that initiate our education, and we may forget that what we know isn't commonly known by all. I am increasingly noticing that the general public has specific positive or negative connotations around the terms carbohydrate, protein, and fat. This is a problem, because all macronutrients are necessary, and in significant amounts. But fad diets teach us to manipulate them, which can cause serious health problems.

As I write this section, I am in Chattanooga, Tennessee, finishing up the last bits of this book before I hand it over to my editor. Last night during dinner at my hotel, I got into a nutrition conversation with my server. She mentioned her desire to quit smoking but expressed concern that she would start eating everything in sight. How should she quit smoking, she wondered, when she is already trying to quit carbs? Well, indeed that would be a problem—because quitting carbs and quitting smoking are both surefire ways to feel irritated. We discussed ways to kick the cigarette habit, all while including carbs in her diet as part of the plan. Our conversation—and so many others like it that I've had with people over the years—points up the intense confusion surrounding nutrition choices that is so commonplace in our culture today. I even see and hear about children in school lunchrooms eating only high-protein foods because they say it is "healthy," or at least that's what their parents have told them. We've picked up so much bad information from fad diets, and we are in turn passing it on to our children. And that bad information so often relates to the macronutrients that make up most of what we eat.

Macronutrients are an important part of our diet, so let's not make drastic changes that eliminate entire macronutrients. We must take the negative connotations off of foods, and focus on including all of them in all of our meals.

Goal

Have you fallen prey to vilifying one of the macronutrients? Try this:

Use the ChooseMyPlate.gov figure (included earlier in this chapter) as a guide, and start by trying to make one meal per day fit with that diagram. Flavor the foods in each of those categories as you like. Your vegetable may be tossed in olive oil (which will contribute to the macronutrient of fat as well as providing a heart-healthy MUFA). Your dairy may be cheese or yogurt you use in the recipe for your grain or protein. Be flexible and think creatively!

Meal Planning

As we cover some of the most common nutritional glitches, you may notice a theme: planning. The good news is that proper planning can become a solution to many wellness pitfalls. With some good management techniques, we can improve the actual nutrition content of our meals—provided we are making sure to eat meals!

For many of us, meal planning is a dreary chore. But attitude makes all the difference (and I am talking to myself here!). If we think of meal planning as dreary, it definitely will be. However, if we consider it a fact of life and decide to make the best of it, then it may change the results. And having a plan can feel amazing. Focus on how great it's going to feel when we don't have to figure out every meal on the fly, worrying about it all day long.

When I discuss meal planning with clients, the biggest difference between my advice and their experiences are the expectations. Most people try to institute meal planning on too big a scale. The plan tends to encompass cooking a fresh, brand-new dinner every night, packing lunch ahead for every day, and making an elaborate breakfast each morning. This is generally not realistic or necessary. For one, most meals will have leftovers, and one night's dinner will provide for a smorgasbord dinner another night. And not every dinner has to be extravagant. Keep a couple of low-key ingredients on hand that can be quickly assembled if you're running late or skipped if last-minute activities arise.

The secret is to build your meal plan around your busy life, and that includes planning for the plan to fall apart! Here are some steps to consider:

o   Review your weekly calendar and your responsibilities for the upcoming week. Is it business as usual, or could certain activities interfere with typical meals or time to cook?

- o Decide to pick a focus: breakfast, lunch, or dinner. Planning for all the meals may be a bit much, especially if you have already set some other nutritional goals. Remember: we want to make just a few changes at a time.

- o Recognize that even the best-made plans can be broken. We cannot predict all circumstances. With that in mind, consider your plan B. I encourage my clients to keep ingredients on hand for a quick mindless meal that you can throw together, as well as to always have a portable snack available in case a planned meal gets missed.

Goal

Do you want to be and feel more successful at meal planning? Begin here:

Starting with the three tips above, pick a day to sit down with your calendar, choose two or three meals you want to plan for the week, and devise specific ideas for them.

Vitamin D and Calcium

For the average healthy adult, the main micronutrients that tend to be lacking in the diet are vitamin D and calcium. Why is this? Vitamin D is not found naturally in a lot of foods. The foods that are fortified in vitamin D (meaning that it has been added to a food that doesn't naturally contain it) tend to be consumed less frequently by adults. One of the main sources I am referring to is milk. Milk is also a main source for calcium, and your body needs vitamin D to absorb calcium.

Another way we get vitamin D is by synthesis in the skin from UVB sun exposure. When wearing sunscreen, this synthesis is inhibited. This can really feel like a catch-22, since we know that sunscreen is important for prevention of skin cancer. The amount of strong UVB rays that can both reach the earth and help with vitamin D synthesis is diminished in parts of the world with higher latitudes.

If you do need to take vitamin D as a supplement, it is important to have it with a meal, preferably one containing enough fat, because vitamin D is a fat-soluble vitamin. Many people taking supplements do not realize the importance of taking them with the right foods to enhance absorption.

Review your typical food intake, and look for sources of vitamin D and calcium. Vitamin D levels below 20ng/mL (nanograms per milliliter) are considered a deficiency by the Endocrine Society, and levels between 21 and 29ng/mL as an insufficiency. Levels above 30 have better health outcomes, and levels above 50ng/mL are said to decrease incidences of colon cancer.

Goal

Do you know if you are getting enough vitamin D?

Have your vitamin D checked at your next visit to the doctor. It can't hurt to know your number.

Seasonal Foods

We cover a lot of nutritional ground when we embrace the value of seasonal foods. To begin with, the taste of in-season foods is superior. And when food tastes better, we are more likely to eat it. We also don't have to do as much to a seasonal food to prepare it or improve its taste. For example, if you have strawberries in the Midwestern United States in June, they will be juicy, sweet, and delicious right off the bush. If you buy them in the Midwest in December, they've been picked much earlier and then shipped from a faraway warm country. They are going to need some added sugar to cut the tartness.

Seasonal foods also have the benefit of freshness. When a food is seasonal and local, it's bound to be fresh, which means fewer preservatives and preservation techniques have been employed, and you ultimately have a less processed product. One of the easiest ways to eat seasonal foods is by buying local. And that creates a win-win situation for your community. Buying local has an intrinsic economic value and keeps the food cycle going: we end up getting more variety and quantity, with improved quality and process along the way.

Goal
Would your diet become more diverse and tasty by incorporating more seasonal foods? How about focusing on fruits and vegetables?
Make a list of the seasons, and all the local fruits and vegetables in your area that fall under each. Keep the list out to easily reference, and see if you can buy and prepare two to three fresh seasonal foods per week.

Ditch the Scale

I've recommended Ditching the Diet, and I advise you to do the same with your scale. If you tend to weigh yourself regularly, it really is a habit that is valuable to break. Seeing a number on the scale is not what is holding you to healthier eating. It is what is making you feel bad about yourself. Scale watching is a shame technique and not motivating. It promotes the negative stories we tell ourselves about who we are. The scale needs to go, and the stories must change.

About six or seven years ago, I stopped by a friend's office in the middle of the day for a quick hello. As she approached to meet me at the door, I said, "Hey, you look so cute today!" Her reply was a disgusted scowl, eye roll, and a noise that can best be described as guttural growl. I reacted with a dumbfounded "What?" "Well," she went on to say, "I thought I looked cute today too, so cute that I figured I must have lost weight, so I went straight to my scale and weighed myself. And I am up three pounds! I am so mad because I have been so good about working out, and I really thought I looked good. I was in a great mood. Now I'm just mad, and it ruined my day."

This interchange may sound familiar to you, because it may echo some of your own experiences and thoughts after stepping on the scale. The psychological effects of weighing are one reason not to do it, but let's go over some other reasons why weighing can do more harm than good:

o More times than not, the scale is a negative influence. The power of perceptions about our weight is immense, and can be used to build us up or tear us down.

o Using weight as the standard by which to measure healthy behavior changes is a poor and inaccurate gauge.

o Weight can fluctuate by multiple pounds from day to day for factors unrelated to a gain or loss in fat mass.

o Muscle weighs more than fat but takes up less space and is more metabolically active. With an increase in regular exercise, weight may fluctuate up within a body that is slimming down because metabolism is burning more calories.

o Knowing our weight is not necessary for keeping healthy behaviors in check. It may in fact send you careening toward the pastries, since it makes you think all the work you're doing isn't working.

Sometimes we hear that regular weighing can help us make healthier choices. If the scale is going up, it reminds us that we need to get back on track. I would argue that this probably works for only a handful of people, and that the exact same process can take place without weighing ourselves. We know when we have been overindulging and eating poorly. We know when our clothes are fitting a little more snugly. That is enough information to adjust some of our habits and be mindful about various behaviors. We can make a slight correction without ever having to weigh ourselves to confirm the suspicion. The confirmation isn't necessary, and may do more harm than good. For recovering dieters, weighing is one way to go straight back into the Dieting Trifecta, because it tempts them to try any fad or food restriction to get those pounds off quickly.

Goal

If you make a habit of weighing, I encourage you to try this scale fast—and fast!

> *If you can't bear to throw away the scale, begin by moving it to a hard-to-reach place where you won't lay eyes on it readily. Instead of thinking about your weight, focus on other goals you have set, and track your progress on the Ditch the Diet Habit Tracker found in the back of this book.*

Eat at Home

I love eating out. I have a magnet that says "I'd rather make reservations," and on many days that is the honest truth! Deciding what to prepare for a family of five every day can beat me down. But eating at home more often is a simple goal that can help some of the health challenges we face. There are so many interferences at restaurants that can throw off our nutritional game. Even if we have healthy ways to avoid the pitfalls of eating out, these moving parts can overcomplicate things when you are trying to create new habits in your life.

Let's consider a few of the obstacles we face when eating out:

o **Portion size:** One size fits all in a restaurant, despite the fact that people require different amounts of food at different times.
o **Ingredients:** Restaurant food tastes good for lots of reasons, and sometimes it is because the food is full of more delicious fat and sugar than you may use in a similar dish prepared at home.
o **Limited choices:** You may be in the mood for a salad or something light when all that is offered on the restaurant menu is burgers and fries. You may welcome that food some days, but the days that you are craving health, try to get it!

I relate to the appeal of eating out, yet the behaviors involved in eating at home will set us up for improved health on multiple levels. Grocery shopping and meal planning may not be perfected overnight, but are valuable skill sets that contribute to the healthy lifestyle you crave. You will have a greater variety of foods available in your house, which helps you eat healthier and enjoy it too. When preparing a meal at home, you have more control over the ingredient list. The practice of eating meals together as a family has also been shown to have both physical and psychological benefits. For children, some of those benefits include not only a healthier diet, but also better academic performance, decreased use of alcohol and drugs, and closer relationships with parents. Have I convinced you yet?

Contrary to popular perceptions, eating at home does not require you to be a master chef or have extra time. Some of the best meals can be pulled together quickly and simply. Though it may feel a little cumbersome at first, as you begin to change your habits you'll find that cooking in can be more enjoyable than you ever realized. And, when choices at home are limited, there is always cereal!

If you do eat out—and we all do—try this tactic for a healthier approach. Ask for a to-go box to come with your meal. Place a portion in the box at the start, so you have an automatic stopping place and can assess satiety and fullness. If you are still hungry once you've finished what's on your plate, get more bites from the box. Whatever is left becomes a meal for later.

Goal

Do you want to tackle cooking and eating at home more often? Try this strategy:

Come up with four dinner plans (new, or old faithfuls), and create a plan to prepare one per week. If you live with others, plan the meal around everyone's schedules so that you can eat together. Once you've mastered this, up the ante to two meals, or three.

Food Journal

Keeping a food journal can be a valuable tool. Even logging what you eat one day per week has been shown to improve food intake, meal planning, and overall healthy eating habits. It is not necessary to record everything we eat every single day, nor is it necessary to measure every food. Simply try keeping a food journal for one to three days periodically, or even one day a week for a couple of months. This will allow you to get a feel for what and when you are eating during the day, the portions you typically eat, and what those portions look like on your plate—all of which will point to common patterns or habits you may have.

This moderate form of food journaling will give you an opportunity to work on mindfulness with your eating. Excessive food journaling can be counterproductive when it comes to eating mindfully because it is easy to slip into a good-versus-bad mentality and ignore some of our own cues in deference to what we think we "should" be eating. So, the goal of food journaling must be practiced with the same moderation used with our other nutritional goals. When you are journaling, remember everything you have learned in the foundation levels of the Pyramid to Healthy Eating: eating mindfully, allowing yourself to eat, accepting your body, and building lasting habits.

What is the best method for keeping a food journal? Since the journal is meant to give you information and complement your other healthy habits, several key elements are important:

- o **Measure properly.** Use measuring cups designed both for dry and liquid ingredients, a scale for measuring grams and kilograms, and pour food and drinks into the plates, bowls, and glasses that you typically use. Since you will be eating mindfully, you may find that you want more or less than you prepared, and you can adjust measurements accordingly as you progress. You now have an idea of how much you typically eat, and what it looks like in your dishes.
- o **Record the times that you eat.** This can give you insight into why you might be so hungry at 10 a.m. every day, or why you crave a candy bar at 3 p.m. It may also alert you to a newly developing habit, such as eating late at night.
- o **Record specific brands of packaged foods.** If you have questions about ingredients that are in a particular product, this provides a reference point. This information can be particularly useful if you suspect food intolerances or sensitivities.
- o **Record all food and drinks.** It's so easy to omit random snacks. And people commonly forget to include drinks, though they are important parts of the big picture.

Once you get good at journaling, here are a few additional elements you might choose to include in your food journal.

- o **Hunger/satiety scale:** This scale can be in the form of a rating system to determine how hungry you are when you sit down to eat, and then how full you feel at the end of the meal. On a scale of 0 to 10 with 0 being not hungry at all, and 10 being stuffed, try recording a number at the beginning and end of every food or meal encounter. This can be a useful tool to teach yourself to be a mindful eater.

o **Food/mood scale or notation**: This scale can be as simple as recording how you are feeling when you sit down to eat. You can also add how you feel after the meal as well.

o **Symptom diary:** This is helpful for people suffering from possible food-related intolerances, whether they know if a food is causing the symptoms or not. As a dietitian working with many people diagnosed with IBS, I find this bit of information in the food journal particularly helpful.

Goal

If you think keeping a food journal would be helpful for you right now, try this:

Use the food journal template in Appendix F, or another journaling medium of your choice, to keep track of what you eat for three days. Consider how this practice may impact your knowledge of and attitude toward your own nutritional health.

Sugar

Sugar has to be a topic for discussion in this chapter, because it is about to be the new gluten, if it's not already. That is, sugar is getting unilaterally stricken from diets as if it is pure evil. Yet sugar, like every other food, has its place in our diet. It adds value not only by making things taste good, but also by serving as the building block of carbohydrates, our primary energy source. Of course, as with any food, if we overdo it, then some of its value is diminished. And at certain amounts, sugar can certainly become unhealthy.

But sugar is not in and of itself bad, whether it occurs naturally in a food or is artificially added. A food can have sugar added to it, and still boast its innate value. A sweet honey dressing on top of a salad doesn't take the fiber, vitamins, minerals, and phytonutrients out of the salad. It enhances the flavor, probably making you more likely to eat it! And how about all the foods that naturally contain sugars, such as milk, yogurt, and fruits? Diets that eliminate all sugar would have these eliminated as well, though they contain all kinds of value, including the sugar content!

So what does the evidence say about how much sugar we should have in our diets? When we talk about sugar in the diet, we tend to focus on "added sugar," the sugar not found naturally in foods. A soda, for example, would be a source of added sugar, as would syrup or the sugar that is found in icing, cakes, and cookies. The 2016 Dietary Guidelines suggest that added sugar can be approximately 10 percent of our total daily calorie intake, or 50 grams (based on 2,000 calories). This is on top of the sugar found naturally in foods (which has already been accounted for in the recommendations that are found using the "Choose My Plate" method we looked at earlier in this chapter). In other words, the grams of sugar found naturally in fruits, grains, and dairy would not be counted as part of the 50 grams/day recommendation.

Sugar intake is taking its toll in the United States in a variety of ways, including the pervasive effects of soda and processed foods and sweets. One soda a day may not wreck your nutritional goals, but soda tends to be a much bigger part of the average American diet. It has, in many cases, completely eclipsed water! The problem with sugar arises when excess soda and processed foods and sweets replace healthy staples. We don't need to treat sugar like a pariah, but we do need to be careful about the effects of convenience foods and quick fixes.

Goal

Have you been harboring some misconceptions about sugar that need to be amended?

> *Look at your typical daily food intake. If you are avoiding all sugar, create a goal to liberalize that, because the act of avoiding all sugar is probably leading to an occasional sugar bender. If, on the other hand, you are a five-a-day soda drinker, revisit the above section on water, and try the goal of adding more water to displace some soda.*

Conclusions

We have covered a lot of material in this chapter, material that I hope will be a helpful resource and antidote to some of the widespread confusion about healthy eating today. Foods and nutrients do not work in isolation. And as much as it can feel like a formulaic science sometimes, the way we eat is an intricate compilation of our body, mind, and intellect, as well as genetics, culture, personal history, and family dynamics—in other words, it's part of our individuality. There is not one exact answer for everyone, but there is a simple truth: eating is intuitive. And eating should be pleasurable most of the time. Keeping those tenets in mind are a great way to gauge some of our decisions about food.

I'm fully aware that this book is just one resource you'll use in your journey toward wellness. As you approach other resources—cookbooks, blogs, magazine articles, or whatever—ask yourself these questions: Does the nutrition advice you are reading about seem plausible and enjoyable? Does it include lots of different foods with options to be prepared in diverse and unique ways? Does it allow for your own autonomy in making decisions based on the individuality of your needs and wants? The answer should be yes to all of these questions.

I also recommend that you seek the advice of a Registered Dietitian Nutritionist in your search for nutrition answers and solutions. RDNs all have our specialties, personalities, opinions, and individual styles, yet the biggest thing we have in common is our credentialing and ethics, paired with a passion for helping people be savvy about nutrition and their health. Read Appendix A in the back of this book for more details about RDNs and what we offer.

In this book, we have covered a lot of topics and internalized some important concepts to climb out of the Dieting Trifecta together. Consider how much more content and relaxed you feel without the oppressive ever-present thoughts of dieting. When you go back to the basics, stop overthinking, and begin listening, then you can truly Ditch the Diet, reclaim your health, and enjoy food. And I sure hope that you do!

Putting It into Practice

Think about where you are in your journey toward a lifestyle that is free from diets, and consider your relationship with food. Write down a few of your thoughts here.

When you are ready to tackle a nutrition goal, choose *one* or *two* of the topics discussed in this chapter. Use the corresponding goals that are provided, or personalize them to make your own goals. (For those who don't know where to begin, I suggest water, food journaling, or breakfast as great places to start.)

Build in Exercise

Affirmation: I am capable.

BUILDING UP TO A GOAL of daily physical activity is absolutely essential. Our body needs a regular routine of cardiovascular exercise, strength training, stretching, and proper breathing in order to put all the pieces of overall wellness and nutrition together. Let's look at how this routine will help your nutritional goals fall into place.

In conversations with my physical trainer friends, we have hit upon an interesting phenomenon. It seems that physical trainers often get clients that "don't want to worry about nutrition, and plan to stay healthy with just exercise." Meanwhile, my clients frequently tell me that they "can't get into a regular exercise routine, and want to stay healthy with just food." As we each explain to our respective clients, health is not a choice of either/or. Exercise and good nutrition do serve different purposes, but both are vitally important and work together. Well-rounded nutrition improves and bolsters exercise performance, just as consistent exercise can make us seek out some of the nutrition we need.

As with all of our habit changes, building in an exercise routine can take time, diligence, and some degree of trial and error. It also should fit in with your lifestyle, personality, abilities, and interests. Let's be honest: exercise is not always fun. It is hard work, and there is usually a certain level of discomfort. Combine that with the added time commitment and the necessity to prioritize it over other important and fun activities, and the urge to skip exercise can be pretty strong. A consistent exercise routine is a tall order, and it is easy to see how people can get deterred.

In this bonus chapter, I offer a few tips on building exercise into your nutritional health. In order to help you find a routine that works for you, I include some questions that I have my clients consider as we come up with a doable exercise plan.

Schedule

We all have busy schedules, and our days already feel full. How on earth do we add one more thing? In particular, how do we add an activity like exercise, which takes a good chunk of time in and of itself, not to mention prep, travel to a specific place, and then showering afterward. This will require a plan. Scheduling is one of the reasons the exercise solution has to vary from person to person. And sometimes it takes experimentation to figure out the best plan for you.

The good news is that there are many different options to choose from: early morning, midmorning, lunch break, after work or school, and late at night. The inconvenient news is that whatever time you choose will require an adjustment to your schedule. If you have tried one or more of these time slots, did any of them seem to work out more or less than another? Or, if you are avoiding a certain time because you are sure it won't work, take another look, because you might surprise yourself! I know that I surprised myself when I experimented with an early-morning exercise routine. If you had told me pre-kids that I would complete all my daily exercise by 6:30 a.m. every day, I would have had a good laugh! I used to love late-night aerobics classes in college and after-work evening runs in my twenties. Nighttime exercise energized me until bedtime, and helped me sleep better once I finally turned out the lights. However, when I tried that same schedule after having my first baby, I was frustrated and disappointed to realize I couldn't make it work like before. It wasn't necessarily a scheduling issue at this point; it was motivation. Because I was more tired at night, I was less motivated to exercise. And with each successive kid, I became less able to keep an evening exercise schedule consistent.

At this current stage of my life, with children ranging from elementary school to high school, both my schedule and my mom duties dictate early-morning workouts. Even on days that my schedule is more flexible and I think a midday workout is feasible, that time slot doesn't work out well for me. It hangs over my head and makes me less productive throughout the hours leading up to it. It also often gets pushed aside in favor of other, more pressing things that come up. In addition, I have found that my emotional strength and willpower are a commodity that dwindles as the day progresses. Apparently, I am not alone in this. In fact, it is widely understood that our mental strength is far greater earlier in the day. And mental strength and willpower are key elements in, first, getting us off the couch and, second, helping us push through the discomfort of a tough workout. Ten years from now, my workout schedule may be completely different. Or, my patterns could be so ingrained that I continue with them just as they are.

I use myself as an example to illustrate how different circumstances can impact even the same person at different stages of life. Now consider how much variation there is from person to person. That's where personality and life circumstances come into play. Here are some questions to consider as you begin thinking about exercise and your personal schedule:

o   What is your work/daily schedule and is it flexible?
o   Do you have a chunk of time in your day when you could have an extended workout, or are there multiple times during the day when you could fit in 10 minutes each?
o   Can you shift your sleep schedule to go to bed earlier and then get up earlier to exercise?
o   Is there a point during the day or evening that is an obviously good time to exercise yet motivation is difficult? How can you overcome that obstacle?

The answer to overcoming motivation obstacles may become clear as you consider some additional aspects related to your personality and life circumstances in the following section.

Personality

If the idea of shaking your booty in a fast-paced Zumba class makes you twitch and sweat, then that may not be the exercise choice for you. On the other hand, if you feel energized and excited at the prospect of dancing your heart out while also getting a good workout, that is the spark you are looking for. Embrace your personality and unique characteristics to find the activities that are perfect for you, and motivation will become easier.

Consider these questions in assessing your activity interests:

o   How do you feel about the outdoors? Are there any outdoor elements that make you uncomfortable?
o   Do you feel confident or shy working out in a gym?
o   Do you like tons of energy, loud music, and someone yelling encouragement, or do you prefer quiet motivation?
o   Do you like working out alone, in a large group, or perhaps with just a buddy or two?
o   Are you highly competitive, and do you enjoy exercise as part of a competitive game or sport?

As you answer these questions, think about activities that fit your needs and preferences. Certain sports such as tennis or Ultimate Frisbee can be a great source of cardiovascular exercise, and a fun addition to a strength-training regimen. Something like taekwondo lessons can provide flexibility, strength, and focus that would nicely complement the additional exercise needs of a runner. There are countless options. Think about what you like and see what ideas you can try in order to establish a plan that works for you.

Life Circumstances

Certain factors out of your control may make specific exercise options more or less feasible, either opening up some opportunities or requiring additional brainstorming. These are just a few questions to make you ponder your own life circumstances, and how they impact your answers in the previous sections:

o   Do you travel frequently? Are there exercise options available at your destinations?
o   Is your neighborhood a safe place to engage in outdoor activities?
o   Do you have any injuries that make typical exercise more difficult or even off-limits?
o   Do you have money to spend on exercise?

All of these considerations should play a part in what form of exercise you choose, and when you choose to do it. There are a plethora of options, so expect to spend some time trying different kinds of exercise to figure out what works for you. If you have tried exercise before and later quit, then reflect on what you might have disliked about that particular exercise routine or what made it difficult to maintain. Use that knowledge to explore new options.

Incorporating routine exercise into your life requires a commitment, and it may even be a little disruptive to life as you know it. It won't always be fun; sometimes it will be just the opposite of fun. However, the long- and short-term benefits of exercise are astounding, and an irrefutable investment in your overall health and your future.

Types of Exercise

According to the Department of Health and Human Services, most healthy adults should get a minimum of 150 minutes of moderate-intensity aerobic activity or 75 minutes of vigorous-intensity aerobic activity per week, plus strength training for all major muscle groups at least two times per week. For additional and even more extensive health benefits, increase moderate-intensity aerobic activity to 300 minutes per week, or 150 minutes of vigorous-intensity aerobic activity. Let's break this down into charts:

MODERATE-INTENSITY AEROBIC ACTIVITY — TIME
150–300 minutes/week = 2.5–5 hours/week = 30–60 minutes/day, 5 days/week

MODERATE-INTENSITY AEROBIC ACTIVITY — TYPE
Walking (very brisk, 4 mph)
Bicycling (light effort, 10–12 mph)
Playing doubles tennis
Mowing the lawn

VIGOROUS-INTENSITY AEROBIC ACTIVITY — TIME
75–150 minutes/week = 1.25–2.5 hours/week = 15–30 minutes/day, 5 days/week

VIGOROUS-INTENSITY AEROBIC ACTIVITY — TYPE
Running or jogging (6 mph)
Hiking
Bicycling (fast, 14–16 mph)
Playing singles tennis
Playing a game of basketball
Playing a game of soccer

These charts show that exercise requirements can be translated into many different, doable variations. You can mix moderate with vigorous activities for even more diversity. Going back to chapter 10 on building lasting habits, it is usually helpful to track your progress when beginning a new exercise regime or mixing up an already established routine. Use the

Ditch the Diet Habit Tracker found in the appendix of this book as a springboard. Write down your exercise plan, and track it as you go. Adjust as necessary, and don't add too many new pieces at once.

Implementing a Plan

When considering a new exercise routine, it is important to take a look at your current status when it comes to activity, fitness level, and overall health. If it has been a while since you were last active, begin by getting the all-clear from your physician. That said, walking is a great starting place for most people. Walking can be as mild or as intense as you choose. For example, for the first few months you can walk short distances along flat routes; or you can walk at a consistently moderate level using hills and speed to add intensity. The key is to make it a routine and find ways to stick with it. You will be more successful sticking with your plan if you first spend time thinking through the questions in this chapter about schedule, personality, and life circumstances, and then build your routine around your answers.

Overcoming Common Pitfalls

Sometimes, changes in life circumstances will cause a once-consistent exercise routine to get pushed aside. You wake up one day and realize you haven't been to the gym in three weeks! Or, instead of exercising four times per week, you realize that for the past month you have exercised just once a week. That's when it is time to reevaluate. Take a look at your current situation, and come up with a list of factors that have sabotaged your routine. If you've been sidetracked by short-term issues like illness, injury, or vacation, you're probably ready to hop back on your plan. Or, if your factors are bigger and more long-term, such as a recent job change or a move to a new city, then you'll need to make some decisions about new exercise times and routines.

I am confident that every person, regardless of their individual limitations, can discover activities and create plans that will work for them. And I know that as exercise becomes part of the fabric of your life, you will notice benefits across all areas which will continue to propel you forward. Press on to reach the goal!

Don't Forget Your Psychological Health

by Kathy L. Sieja, MA, LPC (retired)

Affirmation: I choose love.

WHEN MY DAUGHTER JULIE asked me to share some of the things I learned in my work as a Licensed Clinical Counselor for over 30 years, it was with delight and honor that I wrote this bonus chapter to her book. I believe, as she does, that psychological well-being impacts all areas of our lives. During my years as a counselor in a private practice, I always focused on the issues and concerns of each individual client/patient, but I also addressed some common things each of us can do to improve our psychological well-being. I've summarized my advice here, with specific practices that I believe can lead a person into a healthier way of life.

These aspects of good psychological health are presented in no specific arrangement; that is, I haven't prioritized them in order of importance, because I see all six as vital in balancing your life and lifestyle.

Move Your Body

Though my practice is about psychological more than physical health, I know the importance of doing something every day that will help to strengthen bones, build muscle, and get you breathing hard. I always hesitated to use the word "exercise" because it often turned my clients off; but, as Julie explains in the previous chapter, regular exercise is essential to both psychological and physical health.

We have learned that when you exercise, your body releases chemicals called endorphins. These endorphins interact with receptors in your brain that help reduce your perception of pain while also triggering a positive feeling in your body. Some research has also shown that exercise will increase the neurotransmitter serotonin. Serotonin is the target of many anti-depressants, which are needed in sufficient levels to maintain mood. Another neurotransmitter that is released when you exercise is dopamine, which helps us focus, feel motivated, and stay productive. All of this action in your brain leads to a sense of well-being, improved mood, increased self-esteem, better body image, higher energy levels, improved memory, and sounder sleep. With all that positive stuff, how can someone not want to exercise?

Sleep 7–9 Hours Every Night

So much available research talks of the vital importance of sleep for every single person, and for good reason. For therapists, "How do you sleep at night?" is always a question asked to clients in an initial appointment. Once, when I asked that of a young woman I was seeing, she answered, "Well, I sleep in front and my boyfriend curls around me, kind of like a spoon!" I managed to suppress a giggle and kept questioning, and she eventually shared that she slept quite soundly. More often, my clients told me they didn't sleep well, so I followed up with a more specific line of inquiry: Do you fall asleep easily and wake up often in the night? Or, do you lie there forever waiting to fall asleep in the first place? Or, do you have trouble falling asleep and also wake up for longish periods during the night? All of these possibilities are troubling, and all point to stress/anxiety as the culprit. If we are calm, relaxed, and stress-free, we are more likely to fall asleep and stay asleep for most of the night.

Stress-free sleep isn't always easy to attain, and is relative to so many other things going on in our own situations. Doctors tell us to reduce the stress and stressors in our lives, but we can't just snap a finger and make that happen; we have to work on it—a lot—since there are about a million things that can cause you to feel stress. Here are some considerations for you to evaluate for yourself and your lifestyle.

Speak with your doctor if you have physical ailments that affect your sleep, for instance pain that keeps you awake. An over-the-counter pain reliever or muscle relaxer may help but can have serious side effects if you take it every day for extended periods. If your doctor prescribes sleep medication, be aware that many of these, both prescribed and over-the-counter, can cause dependency if taken every day for a length of time. Such medications are usually meant to be taken as needed, and that means you need to wait until after you have had a sleepless night or two, and then take the medicine so that you can get some rest. It is important that your body learn how to go to sleep on its own, and stay asleep throughout the night.

If you continue to struggle with sleep or even experience only occasional sleeplessness, here are a few options to help you relax:

- o Practice deep breathing like in yoga. Inhale deeply and completely fill your lungs with air. Count one-potato-two-potato; then exhale slowly, completely emptying your lungs. Start over. The key is to focus on your breathing instead of letting your mind wander.
- o Recite the Lord's Prayer or a favorite poem, concentrating on the words.
- o Turn on a light and read until you feel sleepy again. (If you sleep with a partner, you may want to go to another room for your reading.)
- o Try to clear your mind of negative thoughts, regrets, or problems, and think instead of joyful events, beauty in nature, or the loves in your life.
- o Make sure the room is as dark as possible, turn your clock to the wall so the lights don't rouse you, and never have your TV or computer on in the room while you are trying to

sleep. The variegated light from a TV disturbs your brain waves, and the computer figuratively calls your name and will cause your brain to get engaged.

o Consider a sound machine that you can set at a very low volume for a limited time to help lull you to sleep.

Find a solution of your own that will work for you some of the time, bearing in mind that sometimes a tried-and-true solution refuses to do its job correctly, so you may want to branch out to other ideas. Don't wait for your body to rebel on you and make you sick physically or emotionally to get the right amount of sleep. Learn how to sleep longer and better now, before it seriously impacts your health.

Consider Keeping a Journal

Before you shake your head or squinch up your nose—or, worse yet, stop reading—hear me out. You won't know whether keeping a journal is helpful for you until you try it, more than once! Research has told us that writing has a positive effect on the brain, and if you decide to try journaling, you will have personal proof of its benefits (one of which is helping you sleep).

First, let's look at what some of the research has told us about journaling. Neurologically, multiple areas of the brain are co-activated when you write, and this leads to better concentration and focus. But journaling is beneficial in a number of additional ways: it evokes mindfulness, stretches your IQ by increasing your vocabulary, and provides an emotional outlet that is private. Since words represent ideas, as you write your mind is forced to engage in more effective cognitive recall—that is, memory. After writing something down, those ideas become easier to grasp, and we can deal more creatively with difficult issues. Keeping a journal also requires some self-discipline, which leads to confidence and pride of accomplishment.

To start this beneficial activity, here are some tips I've shared with clients over the years:

1. Find a notebook or journal that fits your needs (lined pages or not; spiral-bound or flat; big with lots of space to write or small enough to carry around; perhaps with prompts like Bible verses, inspirational words, or writing ideas). Shop around to find a journal that works best for you. When people ask me if they can journal on the computer, I tell them it's usually best to write with a pen or pencil because your brain has to focus in a certain way to get the words from your mind to your hand; however, if the only way you will write is on the computer, then that is better than not writing at all.

2. Write at about the same time every day. Some people like to write in the morning to start the day on a positive note, especially those folks who build time into the early hours to meditate or plan for the day. The afternoon or evening may also be options, but many find that just before bedtime is the most expedient time for them. If you choose the end of the day, after your bedtime ritual of brushing your teeth and washing your face, journaling can actually help you sleep because it allows you to give your

thoughts, worries, and problems away so that they are no longer on your mind. It doesn't matter when you write, as long as it works enough that you will do it most days.

3. Try to write in the same place most of the time for the same reasons as above. Humans like ritual, and the more we practice something, the better we get at it.

4. Write whatever you want at that moment. It isn't important what you write, but that you write. You may use your journal like a diary and record things you did that day; you may focus on feelings or worries; you might write a poem or draw a picture; or sometimes it may feel right to jot gentle or explosive words all over the page.

5. Keep your journal private unless you choose to share. As a therapist, I never asked my clients to bring their journals to counseling sessions (though sometimes a person would in order to remember what they wanted to discuss). If you are afraid that others will read your journal entries, you may not feel free to write about certain things, so I suggest you find a spot where your journal won't be disturbed by anyone but you.

6. Don't feel compelled to keep journals month after month and year after year, unless you choose to. I had a client who didn't want to keep what she wrote, plus she was afraid others might read it, so she wrote on notebook paper, tore it out of the notebook after writing, and shredded it. She placed a small shredder next to her bed for that purpose, and found that the gentle sound of the shredder actually comforted her.

Try keeping a journal for at least three weeks, at which time you can evaluate how it worked for you. If you got anything at all out of writing, then continue. If you hated it and found that it caused its own kind of stress, then put aside this practice and try again in the future.

Attend to Your Spirituality

In my thinking, spirituality is our own personal way of getting in touch with ourselves and/or a power greater than ourselves. First of all, let's look at the differences between spirituality and religion, as they are very often considered the same thing. Most people worldwide have a belief system that includes God or whatever you call your higher power; often this includes the practice of a religion or worship tradition. For people who deny the existence of a higher power or are confused about what faith is, they can still have modalities of spirituality in which they meditate, relax, or get in touch with nature. All three of these—meditation, relaxation, and connecting to nature—are great no matter your belief system.

In research on spirituality, studies have found that people who consider themselves religious, mindful, or compassionate are more likely to be successful in the following ways: they are happy in their lives and live longer; they have a lower risk of depression or suicide; they are more resilient and more faithful in relationships; they have happier children and are more satisfied with their family lives. One study I read recently stated that spirituality gives people a sense of empowerment, a connection with others, and the ability to cope with everyday life. Another study reiterated that people who practice some kind of spirituality tend to be more gracious, compassionate, optimistic, and able to embrace life's experiences. One of the benefits of regular worship through a religion is that you have a fellowship with other people who believe many of the same things you believe. This can also be true of non-religious people who seek out others with similar views.

Spirituality can bring peace of mind that leads to an overall sense of psychological well-being. How you go about finding that peace is personal. As with the other practices discussed in this chapter, being purposeful and consistent about your worship/meditation/mindfulness can improve your attitude and outlook. Though it's difficult to scientifically define spirituality, we can usually see its benefits in our personal lives.

Socialize Regularly

We know that psychologically, everyone needs to have regular contact with others, and though this is easy for most people, many of us might seek isolation for a number of reasons. Some are embarrassed about how they look or act, and others may find certain people tedious or judgmental. There are times, however, when each of us has specific needs that we cannot satisfy alone, and it helps to have a social network in place when those needs arise.

Socialization helps us develop our own sense of self. Humans cannot live a psychologically healthy life without contact with other humans, although of course some of us need less while some of us can barely get enough. Either way, it is clear that building positive relationships contributes to our overall growth and development. It also enhances our mental functioning, and active communication with someone else can reduce stress and anxiety. This aspect of socialization is proven over and over when we discuss problems with a friend or professional, and almost always feel better after sharing our emotions and receiving spiritual and physical support. This is due in part to the release of those same endorphins that bounce around when we exercise.

In recent years we have also learned that a healthy, active social life can assist in reducing the risk of many physical illnesses; and it can have a preventative effect on age-related cognitive disorders such as dementia. When we inevitably get sick, having a social network can shorten the illness or at least make it easier to bear. Accepting help from others can be difficult for a lot of folks, and reaching out for help even harder, but I guarantee that you will benefit from regular social contact. One of the major symptoms of depression is isolation from others, making it vital to recognize it in ourselves or other people we care about, so that appropriate help can be found.

Feed Your Brain

As I often told my clients, we cannot separate our brains from our bodies, so taking care of one will generally improve the other and vice versa. Most of us can tell the difference in how we feel, think, and behave when we eat healthily, and that is truly the bottom line. You may ask how exactly nutrition contributes to a healthy mind, and I have a few well-documented answers to that question. First of all, restricting foods often results in low blood sugar. And when you Ditch the Diet, consume enough calories from all sources, and eat regular well-rounded meals, that problem can be prevented. We also know that food has a direct correlation to brain functioning, memory, mood, and mental disorders; in fact about 95 percent of serotonin, that feel-good neurotransmitter, is found in our gastrointestinal system. Well-rounded nutrition affects the production of hormones such as endorphins, adrenaline, and thyroid hormones; and when your body is producing the right amount, your brain happily works better. As Julie explains in chapter 11, when you begin eliminating groups of foods, it can often impact a wider range of body systems than intended, and our mental health is one such system.

We sometimes forget to pay attention to our mental health in our everyday lives. We might not recognize that our brains are attached very carefully to our bodies, so when we take good care of one, the other will benefit greatly. The adverse is true as well: if we abuse our body or our mind, the other will suffer. The ancient Hopi Indians of the southwestern part of the United States had a helpful way of thinking about a human. They said that a person is made up of four distinct parts: the head, the heart, the body, and the soul. They knew that the head is important for cognition, making decisions, figuring things out; that the heart is important for dealing with emotions, fairness, and justice; the body is the physical part of us that has to include activity and nourishment; and the soul is our spirit. The Hopis believed that if any one of these four parts is out of whack in some way, then the person cannot and will not function properly. So, if your body has an illness, your cognitive abilities, emotions, and spirit will all be affected by that illness. The same is true for each of the four parts.

In reflecting on the six practices I've recommended here, I should say that, as a therapist, I never asked clients to do things I didn't do for myself. As a child I resented the "do as I say, not as I do" mantra, and so I didn't want to be guilty of not following my own rules. I am certainly not perfect, but I have made it a lifelong habit to practice these six things. Today, in my life as a retiree, I exercise regularly by walking at least three days a week, taking yoga and tai chi classes, and occasionally going to the gym. I eat in a healthy way most of the time, drink lots of water, and try to limit fast food. I have written in a journal most days for the past 30 or so years, sleep pretty well without medication, and have an active social life full of family and friends. I attend to my spirit by practicing my faith, worshipping regularly, and meditating. Of course, I fall short some of the time and often blatantly ignore my own philosophy, but generally speaking, I'm a happy, flawed person. As a result, I feel qualified to help you and others try to get the most out of your life, find the happiness we all seek, and be a productive, active individual who will be good to yourself and give back to others.

Appendices

Appendix A
Where to Find Good Nutrition Information

WHETHER YOU'RE LOOKING for a local expert in nutrition to meet with or researching nutrition advice on the Internet or in books, it is important to know what various credentials mean attached to someone's name. A registered dietitian (RD), also called a registered dietitian nutritionist (RDN), is a healthcare professional recognized as the specialist in nutrition. When you see the designation of RD or RDN, that means the person has a comprehensive education in nutrition sciences as well as supervised experience in all nutrition disciplines, and has passed the rigorous national credentialing exam.

A Registered Dietitian Nutritionist has a very robust educational background in food and nutrition, including college degrees with courses that study the human body and the impact of food and nutrition on health. RDNs have an expertise that make them a uniquely qualified source for nutrition recommendations and advice. Not only do they have a solid grounding in science, but their diverse skill sets tend to make them excellent counselors as well as problem solvers for healthy nutrition practices. In order to maintain credentialing, RDNs are also held to high ethical standards, standards in which providing quality healthcare is the objective.

Just as doctors specialize in specific areas of medicine, so do RDNs. Whatever field an RDN chooses—cardiac, pulmonary, pediatric, community, wellness, sports, digestive health, and so on—in order to maintain their registration status they must participate in and complete ongoing continuing education within their specialty and career path. This continuing education must cover areas of nutrition that meet the specific goals for each RDN, even if they choose not to work.

Providing quality healthcare is a multidisciplinary endeavor requiring a whole host of professions to meet people's needs. Physicians obviously provide a big component of our healthcare needs. However, nutrition is not their specialty, and they depend upon RDNs for this expertise, just as we depend upon doctors for their unique expertise. Unfortunately, anyone can promote a 500-calorie weight-loss diet using whatever mix of foods they think will sell. It may be a random Internet quack, a popular movie star, or even your family physician, which becomes especially tricky because we lend more credibility to our doctors. Don't be afraid to investigate more closely and stay proactive in your own healthcare.

The objective of this material is to point out the importance of knowing about the person supplying the nutrition information. Many of the people providing nutrition advice, writing books, and opening weight-loss clinics do not have the credentials, the expertise, or the accountability of ethical standards that an RDN is held to. Know your sources, check credentials, and use some of the warning signs listed at the bottom of the Evolution of a Dieter diagram in the front of this book to gauge whether nutrition advice is sound.

Appendix B
Stress Breakers

- o Go for a walk
- o Exercise to work off steam
- o Write a letter to a friend
- o Jot down thoughts in a journal
- o Play some favorite music
- o Water your plants
- o Work in the garden
- o Rearrange the furniture
- o Clean out a closet or drawer
- o Call a friend
- o Work on a craft
- o Take a hot bath
- o Practice a daily relaxation technique
- o Sew, build, paint, or fix something
- o Go to a movie
- o Play with children
- o Dance in your room
- o Talk about your troubles in the mirror
- o See a counselor
- o Visit a place of worship
- o Meditate
- o Write poetry
- o Watch an educational show on TV
- o Wash your car
- o Make a list and set priorities
- o Say no to three things
- o Tell someone what you really need
- o Get a massage
- o Take some quiet time for personal reflection

Appendix C
Mantras/Affirmations

- o   I am worthy
- o   I can choose positive thoughts
- o   I surround myself with loving people
- o   I am enough
- o   I respect the wisdom of my body
- o   I am strong
- o   I value progress, not perfection
- o   I am beautiful right now
- o   My body does not determine my self-worth
- o   Happiness is beautiful
- o   I am thankful for my body and what it can do for me
- o   I am capable
- o   Strong mind means strong body
- o   I can listen to my body
- o   I am authentic and uniquely me
- o   My eyes reflect the beauty of the world around me
- o   I am confident in my decisions
- o   I am allowed to take up space
- o   My body is mine and mine alone
- o   I love myself
- o   I am more than this
- o   I was made for this
- o   I am worthy of love
- o   I am not a problem to be solved
- o   I can do hard things
- o   My body is wise and my intuition is strong
- o   My mind is clear and open
- o   I am strong, I am beautiful, I am enough
- o   I enjoy lots of different foods
- o   I choose love

Ditch the Diet 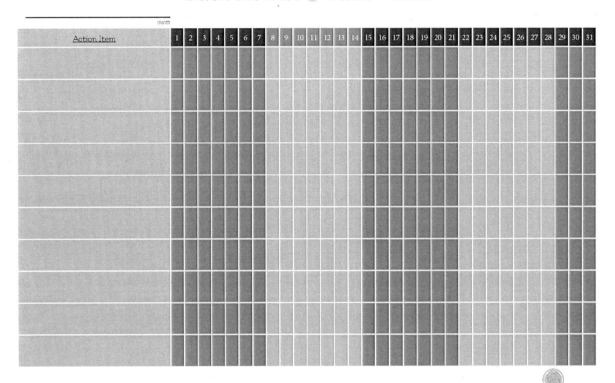 Habit Tracker

month

Action Item	1	2	3	4	5	6	7	8	9	10	11	12	13	14	15	16	17	18	19	20	21	22	23	24	25	26	27	28	29	30	31

Ditch the Diet ● Habit Tracker

month _____

Action Item	1	2	3	4	5	6	7	8	9	10	11	12	13	14	15	16	17	18	19	20	21	22	23	24	25	26	27	28	29	30	31

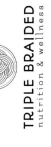

TRIPLE BRAIDED
nutrition & wellness

Appendix E
Overnight Oats and Acai Bowls

Overnight oats, generally eaten cold, are a unique and fun alternative to oatmeal. There are many variations on how to make them. Included here is a basic recipe we use and love at Triple Braided.

Acai [ah-sah-ee] bowls, as we make them, are basically thick smoothies topped with all sorts of delicious goodness that you eat with a spoon. It's a great way to get a fruit or two in at breakfast along with some added protein and carbohydrates.

Overnight Oats (1 serving)

½ cup old-fashioned rolled oats
½ cup milk or unsweetened almond milk
¼ cup regular or Greek yogurt (optional)
½ tablespoon chia seeds
1 tablespoon maple syrup
Pinch of salt
½ teaspoon vanilla extract

Add all ingredients to a container with a sealing lid or a mason jar, mix together, and put in the refrigerator overnight. Top with fresh fruit in the morning and dig in. Favorite fruit toppings: raspberries, strawberries, green apples, bananas, blueberries, pomegranate seeds.

Acai Bowls (1 serving)

1–2 cups frozen fruit (any mixture of banana, blueberries, mango, peaches, berries)
6 ounces regular or Greek yogurt
2–4 ounces cranberry, orange, or pineapple juice (or use milk or water if preferred)

Add all ingredients to a blender and mix until smooth. Pour into a bowl and top with any or all of the following: whole fruit, granola, chia seeds, toasted almonds, pecans, walnuts, honey, cocoa nibs, ground flaxseed.

Appendix F
Food Journal

Date and Time of Meals and Snacks	What I ate and drank	My serving size

References

Duhigg, C. 2014. <u>The Power of Habit: Why We Do What We Do in Life and Business</u>
New York: Random House.

The Institute of Medicine, Food and Nutrition Board, National Academies. *Acceptable Macronutrient Distribution Ranges.* Retrieved May, 2017, from ncbi.nlm.nih.gov

Satter, E. (2018). Ellyn Satter Institute. ellynsatterinstitute.org

Steinem, G. 2016. <u>My Life on the Road </u>New York: Random House

United States Department of Agriculture. *Choosemyplate.gov.* Retrieved April 2017, from choosemyplate.gov

U.S. Department of Health and Human Services and U.S. Department of Agriculture. *2015-2020 Dietary Guidelines for Americans.* 8th Edition. December 2015. Retrieved May, 2017, from health.gov/dietaryguidelines/2015/guidelines

U.S. Department of Health and Human Services, Physical Activity Guidelines Advisory Committee. *Physical Activity Guidelines.* Retrieved January 2018, from health.gov